Understanding Leaky Gut & Hormones for Women Health 2 Books In 1

SIMPLE STEPS TO AVOID COMPLICATIONS, REDUCE MEDICAL EXPENSES, DECREASE STRESS AND LIVE A HEALTHY & PROACTIVE LIFE

DR. ASHLEY SULLIVAN, PHARMD

Copyright © [2024] by [Dr. Ashley Sullivan, PharmD]

All rights reserved.

No portion of this book may be reproduced in any form without written permission from the publisher or author, except as permitted by U.S. copyright law.

Understanding Leaky Gut & Digestive Health

Simple Steps to Avoid Complications, Reduce Medical Expenses, Decrease Stress and Live a Healthy & Proactive Life

Written By Dr. Ashley Sullivan PharmD

Contents

Introduction	#
1. The Marvels of Digestion	#
2. Unraveling Digestive Disorders	#
3. The Gut-Brain Connection	#
4. Nourishing Your Digestive System	#
5. Lifestyle Choices for Digestive Wellness	#
Revitalize 360	#
6. Healing Herbs and Remedies	#
Help Transform Lives	#
7. The Impact of Gut Health on Skin and Immunity	#
8. Digestive Health through Life's Stages	#
Real Stories of Gut Transformation	#
Conclusion	#
Share the Knowledge	#

Gut Friendly Recipes   #

Medications for Digestive Disorders   #

References   #

Introduction

As a child, I waged a relentless battle against my mother's attempts to conquer my aversion to vegetables and fruits. She tried a million different ways to get me to eat healthy food. I remember her saying, "You are what you eat," which often left me feeling confused. I questioned how on earth I could transform into a carrot or an apple simply by ingesting them. Perhaps you too have memories like this from your youth. Yet, even amidst my protests, my mother's recurring mantra remained an echo in my ears. Little did I know that over the years this seemingly simple phrase would unveil its profound truth.

Through a journey marked by trial and error, I discovered a revelation that transcends the whimsical notion of turning into a vegetable. I realized that we truly "are what we eat" because our gut only functions fully when it is fed well. The key then to a flourishing life lies in nurturing our gut—the epicenter of vitality.

In this book, I invite you to explore the transformative power that resides within the delicate ecosystem of our gut. Unveiling the secrets to fortifying it not only enhances our immune system but also acts as a catalyst for overall physical and mental well-being. Join me as we delve into the captivating world of gut health, where every morsel we consume becomes a brushstroke on the canvas of our inner vitality. It's time to repaint the story of our health, to embrace the symbiotic blending of our food and our gut.

Sandra's Story

Struggling with gut health has become extremely common, especially for women in middle age and above. I often see this both in my functional medicine practice and in my health coaching clients. Sandra, a forty-two-year-old woman, was caught in the whirlwind of life's demands, a familiar narrative for many women in middle age and beyond. As she navigated the challenges of being a devoted mother of three, her days were marked by the relentless grind of stressful, long work hours.

Sandra's demanding routine had become a breeding ground for chronic stress, a silent but potent disruptor of her gut health. The stressors in her life, stemming from both the responsibilities of motherhood and the pressures of her professional life, cast a shadow on her overall well-being. The impact of stress on her gut health was profound, as it triggered a cascade of physiological responses that threatened to compromise the delicate balance of her gut microbiome.

During this chaotic existence, Sandra found solace in quick, easy, and highly processed food options, further exacerbating her struggle with gut health. The convenience of these choices, while offering a momentary reprieve from her demanding schedule, set the stage for a host of digestive issues. Over time, the constant consumption of processed foods took a toll on her gut, leading to frequent stomach aches and discomfort.

As Sandra battled with her declining physical health, her mental well-being began to crumble under the weight of these stressors. This is because the intricate connection between the gut and the brain, often referred to as the gut-brain axis, plays a pivotal role in regulating mood and emotional responses. The turmoil in Sandra's gut health had started to manifest in her mental state, contributing to a decline in her overall mood and cognitive function.

Not only was Sandra's physical and mental health at stake but her family also began to witness the toll these struggles were taking on her life. Concerned for her well-being, they witnessed a woman they loved grappling with the complex interplay between stress, gut health, and mental health.

The repercussions extended beyond the realms of stress and gut health, reaching into Sandra's cardiovascular system. The chronic stress, coupled with poor dietary choices, resulted in elevated blood pressure levels. The intricate connection between gut health and blood pressure became evident as Sandra's physiological responses to stressors contributed to hypertension.

Sandra's story is an illustration of the intricate web woven between stress, gut health, and blood pressure. It reveals the importance of addressing the root causes of gut-related issues to achieve holistic well-being. Sandra's journey unveils the profound impact that lifestyle stressors can have on our body's intricate systems, which emphasizes the need for a comprehensive approach to health.

Jenny's Story

Next, we meet Jenny, a thirty-nine-year-old woman whose life took an unexpected turn when she found herself seeking care due to persistent stomach aches and bloating. A once vibrant and energetic individual, Jenny's complaint unveiled a cascade of health concerns that had insidiously crept into her daily life.

For several weeks, Jenny battled the discomfort of constant stomach aches and the frustrating sensation of bloating, both of which had become constant companions, overshadowing her ability to enjoy a proper meal. The toll on her physical appearance was evident. She had lost a significant amount of weight in an alarmingly short period, and her skin, once radiant, now bore premature wrinkles.

The impact wasn't merely skin-deep; Jenny's vitality was depleted, and lethargy became her unwelcome companion. Daily activities that were once second nature now became a huge effort, leaving her fatigued and drained. The vibrant woman who once effortlessly navigated her routine found herself grappling with a new reality, one that seemed to age her beyond her years.

As the symptoms persisted, so did Jenny's concern. Each passing day brought new worries, and the confusion around her declining health fueled her anxiety. Her apprehension intensified as her inability to carry out daily activities at an average pace increased, creating a perpetual cycle of physical discomfort and mental distress.

Jenny's journey, like Sandra's, also speaks to the intricate relationship between gut health and overall well-being. Her stomach aches and bloating are not just isolated symptoms; they are windows into a deeper imbalance within her gut microbiome. The repercussions extend far beyond mere digestive discomfort, permeating into her appearance, energy levels, and daily functionality.

As Jenny embarked on the path to seeking care, we peeled back the layers of her struggles to reveal the interconnectedness of gut health with various facets of our lives. It serves as an important reminder that the symptoms we experience are often manifestations of a broader health narrative. Jenny's story speaks to the importance of addressing gut health for a holistic and rejuvenated life.

Claire's Story

Let's delve into the life of Claire, a forty-seven-year-old woman whose health journey began when she found herself grappling with stomach ulcers that defied conventional treatment. The chronic nature of her condition weighed heavily on her, creating a deep sense of distress and concern for her overall well-being.

Claire, the accomplished director of a bustling marketing agency, unfolded a narrative woven with relentless work hours. Her daily grind extended between ten and fourteen hours, demanding her attention at least six days a week. In the chaotic rhythm of her professional life, convenience took precedence over nutrition. Claire found herself relying on processed foods and frequently resorting to fast food options and takeout meals, subjecting her stomach to a barrage of challenges.

This demanding professional life was not the sole contributor to Claire's health predicament. Her sedentary lifestyle, devoid of any form of physical activity, cast a shadow on her well-being. The consequence was evident—Claire found herself teetering on the brink of obesity, a stark manifestation of the toll her work-centric routine had taken on her body.

As her stomach ulcers persisted, so did the emotional turmoil within Claire. The realization that conventional medications were falling short of alleviating her condition heightened her anxiety. Concerns about her health began to permeate every facet of her life, adversely affecting her professional achievements and personal happiness.

Claire's story is a stark reminder of the complex dance between lifestyle choices, gut health, and overall well-being. The ulcers in her stomach were not isolated incidents but rather signals of an internal imbalance exacerbated by her relentless work schedule, poor dietary choices, and lack of physical activity.

As Claire stood at the crossroads of her health journey, the imperative for change became evident. Claire grappled with the urgent need to make amends to her lifestyle. Her symptoms were a call to action, not only to treat her ulcers but to reclaim control over her health and enhance the quality of her life.

In the arc of Claire's narrative, we witness the transformative potential that lies in acknowledging the symbiotic relationship between gut health, lifestyle, and overall well-being.

The Common Denominator

In all three circumstances, the underlying cause was the lack of a healthy, well-functioning gut microbiome (bacterial flora). A common misconception is that eating only green vegetables is the key to "being healthy." However, we need proper nourishment from various kinds of foods to lead an active and healthy life.

More than 60 million people alone in the US suffer from issues related to the gut, such as irritable bowel syndrome and inflammatory bowel disease. Some of these typical issues are bloating, diarrhea, stomach discomfort, gas, migraines, and auto-immune diseases. People have also commonly complained about having mood swings, developing allergies, weight loss/gain, and having food cravings (often related to eating a high processed sugar diet).

When experiencing such issues, people often worry about what they're eating and if eating a certain food will cause their health to worsen. The constant worry and regulation of their symptoms can cause them to have anxiety and mental stress.

Are you going through something similar? Do you feel like you can relate to the symptoms above? Have you also been trying various household remedies and supplements that promise a healthier gut, but to no avail? Are you tired of people giving you unsolicited advice to treat your stomach bloating?

If your response to these questions is "YES," then you have picked up the right book! It will answer all your questions and get you on the proper track to treat your gut.

But how? Well, simply because this book has been carefully researched and thoroughly compiled by me, a practicing pharmacist with a strong interest in holistic and functional medicine. My comprehensive study in medicine has allowed me to understand what type of medicine works best for a particular condition. In addition, I am a wellness advocate and an integrative health coach and have treated people with digestive imbalances. As a female medical practitioner, I have paid particular attention to women who are undergoing digestive issues. These often cause hormone imbalances, particularly when those women have become too lenient with what they are consuming on a long-term basis. With this first-hand knowledge of digestive issues, I intend to empower my readers with knowledge about their digestive system and the importance it plays in their health.

The book is divided into eight chapters. These will thoroughly explain the function of the gut, and the real-life impact when it's not taken care of, helping you to understand the gut's needs and what works best for it, and giving testimonies of people who have had issues with a bad gut and how they were able to treat it with my help.

As I have gathered from my experience, it is exceedingly difficult to achieve the right results unless you have accurate information and methods to do it. So, our journey does not end in gaining more knowledge and understanding; at the back of the book, I have included some delicious and healthy recipes to help maintain optimal gut function.

Join us in this journey of discovery and equip yourself with more knowledge about your gut and digestive system. You can make informed choices on the foods you should eat and changes you can make to your lifestyle. Your future self will thank you for making this investment in yourself. Turn the page and take the first step toward a healthy digestive system!

Chapter One

The Marvels of Digestion

Meet Emma, a vibrant woman in her mid-thirties who is juggling the demands of her paralegal job at a law firm with studying for law exams. One evening, while having dinner, she was blindsided by a sudden bout of severe and persistent diarrhea. Feeling embarrassed and scared, she decided to seek help at the hospital. Little did she know, this was just the beginning of a health rollercoaster.

Soon after, Emma found herself grappling with stomach aches, bloating, gas, and a newfound intolerance to certain foods. Concerned about her health, she embarked on a quest to understand her symptoms, consulting doctors and medical experts. The toll on her energy levels and her ability to complete daily tasks became overwhelming as her health rapidly declined.

A diagnosis revealed Leaky Gut Syndrome, a condition where her intestinal lining had become permeable, allowing toxins and bacteria to escape into her bloodstream. With a tailored diet and medication, Emma reclaimed her health, returning to her routine worry-free and embracing a healthy life once again. Emma's journey highlights the importance of gut health, demonstrating both how it impacts our daily lives and the transformative power of proper care and attention.

Just like Emma, millions of people undergo stomach issues regularly. The reason that it's so prevalent is that most people don't have the required knowledge to diagnose their issues and don't understand the role that our gut plays in maintaining our body. Hence why it's imperative to know how our digestion works and ways to nourish it.

Why is Healthy Digestion so Important?

Food is our body's fuel. We need it to conduct various tasks throughout the day. When food is consumed, the process of digestion breaks it down into a form that can be stored inside the human body.

But what happens when our body is not performing digestion properly? What happens when the food won't break down into a million pieces for digestion?

As we have seen in the featured case studies, we can undergo a multitude of issues that cause hindrances in our daily lives. While it's common to experience some temporary digestive issues occasionally, it's not okay to have these frequently. Some of the recurrent issues I'm referring to are heartburn, diarrhea, constipation, hemorrhoids, gastroenteritis, ulcers, and gallstones. Even though some of these are temporary, they can be quite painful if not treated on time with the proper procedure.

However, sometimes people also develop diseases related to the digestive tissues, which can often remain for a lifetime and prove to be detrimental to health. Some examples are gastroesophageal reflux disease, irritable bowel syndrome, lactose intolerance, diverticulosis, diverticulitis, Crohn's disease, celiac disease, and even cancer. It's crucial to make sure that your gut remains healthy.

But how do we know if our gut is healthy or not? Is there a way to know that?

Overview of the Digestive System

In a healthy digestive system, all the digestive enzymes and juices are produced and used in the right amounts, the good intestinal bacteria are there to be used, the nutrients are absorbed, elimination of pathogenic bacteria occurs, and toxins and waste from the gut are removed. Let's look at a case study of Lindsey to see how an ideal digestive system should be.

Case Study

Lindsey is a thirty-five-year-old accountant who's mastered the art of maintaining a healthy digestive system. She's not your average number cruncher; Lindsey takes a thoughtful approach to her well-being. When it comes to groceries, she's like a detective, meticulously scanning labels so that she can make informed choices to keep sugars and fats in check. Lindsey knows that as she gracefully ages, it's crucial to treat her digestive system with some extra TLC.

Her mornings kick off with a burst of energy, thanks to a thirty-minute yoga session, and she seamlessly integrates gym workouts every two days to stay fit. Lindsey doesn't just balance her books; she's also a pro at managing stress. Recognizing its potential impact on her mental and physical health, she tackles stress head-on, ensuring it doesn't linger.

But that's not all—Lindsey's dedication to digestive health goes beyond the gym. She also keeps a watchful eye on her bowel movements, making sure they maintain a consistent frequency. I want to encourage you that Lindsey's story is an achievable journey of mindful eating, staying active, and managing stress. The advice you'll read in this book can become the blueprint you follow when you begin to prioritize your digestive well-being in the hustle and bustle of everyday life.

Keeping Track of Bowel Movements

You can figure out if all the processes in your gut are being carried out accurately by keeping track of your bowel movements. A healthy person usually takes up to 24-25 hours to completely digest food and expel the waste products from the body. Note the time it took for you to pass out your stool, along with how it looked, to figure out if your body is working properly.

I understand that it can be uncomfortable to talk about the passage of your stool and its appearance, even with a medical practitioner. However, it's important to have this basic knowledge about your stool to check if your gut is working properly.

A normal stool should, ideally, be four to eight inches long, like a log or a cylinder in appearance. If it's coming out in pellets, it's not normal and means that you may have constipation. Conversely, if it's too runny, you have diarrhea. It should look firm and soft. If it was easy to pass out without any major force, then it lies under that description.

In addition, the color of the stool should be brown, with light and darker shades included. Brown is the color of bile, so having a large area of brown is completely normal. If your stool looks green, it's usually okay and can often be because of dietary choices, such as the inclusion of a lot of green vegetables in your food or even the addition of artificial color if it's too green (such as blue cupcake icing!). Medications, such as antibiotics and iron supplements, may also cause green-colored stool. Red, however, can be concerning since it might mean that your colon is bleeding. If you see red in your stool, visit a medical practitioner. Yellow stool is often stinky and can mean that you either have too much fat in your diet or that your food is not being absorbed properly. Whereas a pale white stool can mean that you have some sort of infection.

Moreover, you should only take a few minutes to pass out the stool. If it takes you more than ten to fifteen minutes, it means that you have constipation and lack fiber in your diet. Nutritional sources of fiber include whole grains (brown rice, quinoa, oats, whole wheat bread), legumes (beans, chickpeas, peas), fruit (apples, pears, berries, oranges, bananas), vegetables (broccoli, carrots, brussels sprouts, cauliflower, leafy greens), nuts and seeds, dried fruits, popcorn, and bran cereal. There is no fixed number of times you should be passing stools in a day. It's perfectly normal to pass feces as much as three times a day or as little as three times a week. The essential thing is that you have your own 'normal' pattern of bowel movement.

The Main Organs Involved in the Digestive System

Digestion is a complex process, so before we can talk about how to fix your digestive issues, we need to understand digestion in detail, including how nutrients are absorbed in your body. The main organs that take part are the mouth, esophagus, stomach, pancreas, liver, gallbladder, small intestine, large intestine (colon), and anus. Even before we start eating, the mouth anticipates food, beginning the process of digestion through the creation of saliva and the salivary enzyme known as salivary amylase. This is one of the first enzymes to encounter food as your body begins the process of breaking it down.

Your tongue pushes the food down into your throat, through the esophagus, and into the stomach. The stomach then mixes the food with the various digestive enzymes, until the food is a semi-liquid mixture called chyme. Peristaltic motion helps the mixture slowly release into the small intestine. Once there, the liver, pancreas, and intestines use their digestive enzymes to enhance the process of digestion, readying the food for absorption.

The digestive system is a complex network of nine organs that work together to break down food, absorb nutrients, and eliminate waste. Each organ plays a specific role in this process, ensuring that the body receives the necessary nutrients for energy, growth, and maintenance.

How Does the Gut Absorb Nutrients?

Thousands of small projections lining the small intestine absorb the nutrients, before releasing them into the bloodstream to be used and stored. Water is also absorbed into the small intestine through diffusion into the bloodstream, which is why it's important to drink eight to ten glasses a day to stay hydrated. At the same time, waste products are transferred to the large intestine and into the rectum to be removed.

In addition to the enzymes and digestive juices in the stomach and small intestine, there are gut bacteria called microbes in the large intestine and colon that help to digest food. In total, there are around 100 trillion microbes in your gut, separated into two types: good and bad. The good microbes are known as symbiotic, and the bad bacteria are called pathogens. What we eat determines the benefit or damage our intestine receives. Good bacteria are important in the digestion of macronutrients—like fats, carbohydrates, proteins—and micronutrients, which include vitamins and minerals. After the indigestible nutrients enter the large intestine, the microbes help ferment the remaining proteins and carbohydrates, producing short-chain fatty acids, known as SCFA, which are used as fuel for tasks in the body.

How is Food Digested in the Body?

Let's say you had a chicken sandwich for lunch. Did you get all the basic nutrients for the day? A chicken sandwich primarily includes proteins coming from the chicken, carbohydrates provided by the bread, fiber from any vegetables that might be present in the sandwich, fats from mayonnaise, cheese, butter (or if any oil was used while cooking the chicken), and vitamins, such as vitamins A and B. Proteins are broken down into amino acids, carbohydrates into simple sugars, and fats into glycerol. The different nutrients are broken down by the organs assigned to that task and stored in the body for use in the next few hours of your day.

The carbohydrates found in the bread provide immediate energy, taking only fifteen minutes to three hours to be absorbed. The fat source found in dairy products (mayonnaise and cheese) absorbs quickly into the body, taking between thirty minutes to two hours to be fully digested. Fiber-containing vegetables and fruits, meanwhile, take a while longer (almost a whole day) to be absorbed. At almost three days, the protein source found in the chicken takes the longest to absorb.

Have you ever noticed that eating certain kinds of food causes you discomfort, for example, spicy food? It's because some foods are easily absorbed by the body, giving you proper energy from the nutrients, while some make your digestive system work harder. Spicy food, like hot chili peppers; fatty foods, such as red meat; fried food, such as french fries; and acidic foods are more difficult for the body to absorb. In contrast, chicken, eggs, salmon, sweet potatoes, bananas, and rice are easily digested by the human body. This is why most nutrition should come from lean meats, fruits, vegetables, and whole grains.

How Modern Life Puts Our Digestive System at Risk

Our daily life has become so busy that there's barely any time to put effort into what we eat, and we usually end up eating what is convenient: a meal from a fast-food restaurant or packaged processed food. This unhealthy eating leads us to eventually reduce the diversity of foods we consume. According to a study (McDonald et. al, 2018), people who consumed more than thirty types of plant-based food in a week had a wider variety of microbes in their bodies in comparison with those who didn't. This study shows that it's necessary to diversify your foods because microbes are an essential part of digestion.

Additionally, because our lives have become hectic and spending time on ourselves is considered a luxury, we usually don't find the time and energy to commit to exercising daily. However, physical fitness is important; it not only increases the good bacteria in the gut but also helps elevate mood and decrease stress levels.

We have become too involved in the 'grind' that tells us to keep working without any rest. This causes our stress levels to rise, which in turn increases alcohol consumption and encourages indulging in cigarette smoking. These habits eventually cause the body to get sicker, further increasing the use of antibiotics—a huge contributing factor in the destruction of gut bacteria and, ultimately, the destruction of health.

Not taking care of the gut also means fewer enzymes in the body for digestion. Read on further to see how important enzymes are in the digestive process.

The Role of Enzymes and the Digestive System

What are enzymes exactly, and why are they so important? The simple answer is that enzymes are catalysts that speed up the digestion process, without which food will not be broken down the way it needs to be. Carbohydrates need the enzyme amylase to be broken down, whereas proteins require protease, and fats need lipase.

Enzyme Deficiency

A reduction in these enzymes can hinder proper digestion and cause several enzyme deficiencies, such as food intolerance, digestive issues, poor nutrient absorption, weight gain, a poorer immune system, fatigue and lethargy, anxiety and depression, and skin problems.

People who do not consciously take notice of the food they are eating can often develop enzyme deficiency, in addition to having lower microbes in the body. One example is John, a thirty-eight-year-old engineer who suffers from enzyme deficiency due to a genetic predisposition. This condition has an uncomfortable impact on his digestion, inducing cramps, bloating, and nutrient absorption problems. He has to take certain enzyme supplements to aid in digestion and be very careful about his diet. Some enzyme deficiencies are more common in women than in men, such as lactose intolerance. Women, especially, are at a higher risk of developing osteoporosis than men; hence, they need to get enough vitamin C and calcium.

Some enzyme deficiencies are more prevalent in certain areas. This is known as the cultural enzymatic effect. The prevalence of lactose intolerance, for example, has a geographical variation. Studies have shown that it is more widespread in Asia, Africa, the Middle East, and Latin America. Other regions where milk was made a mandatory part of daily diet several thousand years ago developed lactase persistence due to the prevalence of lactose in their diet, and, as a result, these populations can now absorb lactose easily (Anguita-Ruiz 2020).

The Gut Microbiome

The human gut is inhabited by trillions of microorganisms known as the microbiome, which consists of bacteria, fungi, and viruses. They play a very crucial part in the maintenance of the digestive system and overall physical and mental health, affecting the absorption and even the mood of an individual. Gut microbes can be maintained by diet and regular exercise.

The Importance of a Balanced Gut Microbiome

A balanced gut microbiome is essential for the well-being of the digestive system. It makes sure that digestion is efficient, supports the immune system, and encourages good mental health. It also aids weight management through keeping inflammation under control and increasing nutrient absorption. A good microbiome is responsible for preventing disease development, keeping the gut-brain connection healthy, and maintaining healthy metabolism. Maintaining a balanced gut microbiome is an integral part of having a healthy life.

What are Prebiotics, Probiotics, and Postbiotics?

The three "biotics" work in a cyclic manner. Prebiotics are the source of fuel for probiotics and usually take the form of food we eat, such as apples, asparagus, barley, and wheat. Probiotics are the living bacteria in the gut that feed on prebiotics. And postbiotics, such as butyrate, are what the probiotics produce to help regulate the gut environment, which eventually lowers inflammation in the gut.

Gut Wisdom Challenge!

How Well Do You Know Your Digestive System?

- What is the main function of the small intestine in the gut?

1. Storing food

2. Absorbing nutrients

3. Removing Toxins

- Probiotics are good for your health.

1. True

2. False

- How many microbes are there in your gut?

1. 10 billion

2. 10 trillion

3. 100 trillion

- What's the recommended daily water intake for an adult?

1. 1-2 glasses

2. 4-6 glasses

3. 8-10 glasses

- Which of the below organs is not part of the digestive system?

1. Pancreas

2. Lungs

3. Liver

- How many organs are in the digestive system?

1. 3

2. 5

3. 7

4. 9

- Which of these is a good source of fiber content for the body?

1. Sugary cereal

2. White bread

3. Broccoli

- Is physical exercise necessary to maintain your gut health?

1. Yes

2. No

- What is the process called where food breaks down into a semi-liquid mixture called chyme in the stomach?

1. Digestion

2. Peristalsis

3. Absorption

(Answers: 2,1,3,3,2,4,3,1,1)

I hope this chapter helped you understand your digestive system better. However, we have only uncovered the tip of the iceberg here; the digestive system is much more intricate than this. As we continue reading, we will explore its inner workings and its role in our health.

Now that we know how it all works, what happens if it stops working the way it should? How does our body react then? Read on to find the answers to these questions and more.

CHAPTER TWO

Unraveling Digestive Disorders

So far, 88.99 million lives have been completely altered by digestive diseases, to the extent that they reduced the person's life expectancy. The disability-adjusted life years (DALYs) formula calculates the number of life years lost due to ill-health in comparison with a healthy life span. It ranks digestive issues in thirteenth place as the cause of DALYs globally. Cirrhosis and liver diseases prevail more than others. Geographically, South Asia is disproportionally affected by digestive issues over other regions (Wang et. al, 1990).

These alarming statistics call for us to prioritize our gut health so that we may live a prosperous life. However, we can only treat them once we understand how they affect our gut. This chapter will discuss various gut issues and their underlying causes, symptoms, and possible treatments.

The Main Gut Issues

As the statistics suggest, digestive issues have been increasing at an accelerated rate. Let's take Sara, for example. In her early forties, she was dealing with a hiatal. This is caused by a small hole in the diaphragm, which the stomach then pushes through. She commonly felt heartburn, especially if she had consumed too many spices in her food. She also felt that sometimes her food was coming back up in her mouth. In addition, she also experienced chest pain and difficulty swallowing. Since she was also borderline obese, the increased pressure in her abdomen worsened her condition. She was advised to make amends to her routine, eat healthily, and do some physical exercise to keep the symptoms as minimal as possible. Surgery would be considered if the situation didn't improve.

Jasmine, on the other hand, also a middle-aged woman, had colon polyps, a condition in which cells start forming on the lining of the intestine. Her uncle had colon cancer in his later years, so there was a possibility that this was driven by a genetic predisposition. She used to be a smoker as well, which adds to the risk factors but quit when she realized she was in danger of developing cancer. She will soon undergo surgery to remove the colon polyps before there is any chance that they mature into cancer.

Hiatal hernia and colon polyps are just two of the widespread digestive issues witnessed regularly. The table below highlights more recurrent gut issues, detailing what they are, their causes, the common symptoms observed, and what one must do and avoid reducing further issues.

Digestive issue	What it is	Causes	Symptoms	Do's	Don'ts
Constipation	Unable to pass stool regularly	• Lack of fiber in the diet • Change in routine • Medication side effects • Not hydrated enough	• Stomach cramps • Feeling bloated • Feeling sick • Loss of appetite	• Take 18-30g of fiber a day • Eat fruits and vegetables • Exercise regularly • Take prescribed laxatives	• Eat processed food • Add fiber too fast and in sudden large quantities • Drink alcohol • Consume too much dairy
Diarrhea	Watery stool and frequent bowel movements	• Viruses (Coronavirus, Rotavirus, Norwalk virus, etc.) • Bacteria and parasites (E. coli, Clostridiumoides difficile) • Medications, such as antibiotics • Lactose intolerance	• Stomach cramps • Bloating • Nausea • Vomiting • Fever • Blood in stool • Urgent need to empty bowels	• Drink more water to stay hydrated • Take prescribed anti-diarrheal medicine • Take probiotics	• Eat high-fiber or oily/fatty foods • Workout extensively • Consume alcohol or hot beverages • Eat dairy for a while
Colon Polyps	Cells start lining the colon. They can cause cancer over time	• Change in genes can cause the production of cells even when they are not needed, causing polyps to form • Polyps are nonneoplastic (non-cancerous) and neoplastic (can become cancerous)	Initially, polyps might not show any symptoms. However, the common ones are: • Long-lasting diarrhea or constipation • Blood in stool • Anemia • Abdominal pain • Rectal bleeding • Dizziness	• Eat less meat • Eat more fruits and vegetables • Regular exercise • Lose weight if you're overweight	• Consume alcohol • Smoke • Eat fatty foods
Perianal abscesses / hemorrhoids / fissures	Collection of pus near the anus. While they are very painful, they do not affect the absorption of nutrients. It may be red in color and warm to touch.	• A tear in the anal canal • Sexually transmitted infection • Blocked anal glands • Diabetes, diverticulitis, colitis, being the recipient of anal sex, and pelvic inflammatory disease can increase the risk	• Constant, throbbing pain • Release of pus • Swelling, redness, and tenderness around the anus • Constipation • Fever • Chills • Malaise	• Stay hydrated • Have a sitz bath • Act on your bowel movement urges immediately • Use stool softeners or laxatives (prescribed) • Sleep well	• Eat fatty foods • Become constipated • Increase stress

Condition	Description	Causes	Symptoms	Do's	Don'ts
Lactose intolerance	Inability to digest sugar in milk / dairy.	• Lack of production of enzyme lactase in small intestine • Risk factors include increasing age, premature birth, ethnicity and race (Native Americans, Hispanic, Asians and Africans are more prone), cancer treatments, surgery or disease, and small intestinal diseases)	• Bloating • Gas • Diarrhea • Nausea (sometimes vomiting too) • Stomach cramps (All these occur after consumption of milk or dairy)	• Consume lactose-free dairy products • Eat active culture foods, such as yogurt • Use substitutes for dairy, such as soy milk • Eat more vegetables and fruits to get calcium, such as broccoli, fish, tofu, and soybeans • Take lactase tablets	• Consume high-lactase products, such as cheese or butter in large amounts
Hiatal Hernia	The abdomen and diaphragm get separated by a bulge in the stomach. A small hernia is usually harmless. However, larger ones can cause food and acid to go back into the esophagus	• Changes in diaphragm due to age • An injury in the area • Having a large hiatus by birth • Constant intense pressure on the surrounding muscles from lifting weights, vomiting, or forceful bowel movements	• Heartburn • Pain in chest or abdomen • Acid reflux • Bloating • Shortness of breath • Passing black stool • Blood in vomit • Difficulty in swallowing food	• Eat low-fat dairy • Stay hydrated • Eat smaller and more frequent meals • Eat low-fat meals, such as lean chicken and fish • Add more grains (such as bran and oatmeal), beans, broccoli, and carrots to your diet	• Eat spicy food • Drink coffee • Eat dairy products • Eat fatty foods • Eat onions and garlic (they can cause heartburn) • Eat carbonated drinks • Eat or drink citrus fruits

In addition to the above-mentioned digestive issues, there are several more that are important to know about. As I frequently deal with patients with a variety of issues, I have noticed that certain conditions make people more prone to digestive issues.

Gastroesophageal Reflux Disease

Gastroesophageal reflux is a common disease in which it feels like food and stomach acid are moving out of the stomach through the mouth. In this condition, the person experiences heartburn, acid reflux, and abdominal pain, among other symptoms.

Case Study

Emily dealt with a common pregnancy-related issue—gastroesophageal reflux (GERD), particularly in her second trimester. As the baby's weight increased, the muscles around her lower esophagus did not relax how they needed to, sometimes causing stomach acid to come up to her throat. She constantly felt heartburn, had trouble swallowing, coughed, and felt nausea.

Her symptoms were not too severe, and her condition was easily diagnosed and monitored with diet changes. However, if the acid reflux is to such an extent that it may cause concern for esophageal health, and initial medication fails to work, there might be a need to perform a proper diagnosis using an upper endoscopy and reflux testing. The risk of having GERD increases if you are obese, pregnant, have connective tissue disorders, smoke, have an unhealthy eating routine and diet, and consume too much alcohol or coffee.

How to Manage Heartburn through Lifestyle Changes

Fortunately, GERD can be treated with a change in lifestyle if the symptoms aren't severe. Avoiding fried and fatty foods and carbonated drinks, exercising regularly to keep yourself physically active, and reducing weight if you're overweight, combined with making sure that you stop eating two to three hours before you lie down are ways to prevent GERD. Just following these three tips can be life-changing!

Decoding Your Gastroesophageal Reflux Disease

The different techniques to keep GERD at bay are as individual as the person experiencing them; there isn't one way that works for everyone. Henry, an accountant, had to make a minor shift in his pillow angle, elevating it a little, adjust his diet, and decide to avoid his trigger foods to lessen his GERD symptoms.

Penny, on the other hand, found some low-acid recipes and chose to experiment with those to see if they would help her acid reflux. To her delight, they did.

Molly, a yoga instructor, devised a yoga plan for herself, carefully choosing the postures that would help her stomach. Everyone's lifestyle and risk factors are different; find what works in your life.

Bloating: Causes and Remedies

Abdominal bloating, characterized by discomfort and a sense of fullness in the belly, can arise from various factors, including gas, fluid retention, irritable bowel syndrome (IBS), food intolerances, menstrual symptoms, and infections. While some instances can be self-managed, certain causes may necessitate medical attention.

Most often, though, it's attributed to indigestion or the accumulation of gas. Typically, it's not a cause for concern if it's linked to food consumption, does not worsen progressively, and resolves within a day or two.

Common causes encompass:

- *Gas:* The build-up of gas in the stomach and intestines manifests as symptoms like frequent burping, excessive gas, and an urgent need for bowel movement. Triggers may include specific foods or the ingestion of air.

- *Indigestion*: Discomfort or pain in the stomach, possibly accompanied by bloating, commonly results from overeating, excessive alcohol intake, or certain medications.

- *Infection:* Stomach infections, indicated by bloating in conjunction with symptoms like diarrhea, vomiting, nausea, and stomach pain. Bacterial or viral infections may be contributing factors.

- *Small Intestinal Bacterial Overgrowth (SIBO):* Imbalance in gut bacteria leading to chronic symptoms like bloating, frequent diarrhea, and challenges in digestion and nutrient absorption.

- *Fluid Retention:* Triggered by factors such as the consumption of salty foods, hormonal fluctuations, or food intolerances, resulting in heightened fluid retention. Persistent fluid-related bloating may signal underlying concerns like liver or kidney issues.

- *Food Intolerances:* Bloating may ensue after the consumption of specific foods, as seen in lactose intolerance, gluten intolerance, or celiac disease. Eliminating the problematic food source can alleviate symptoms.

In instances where bloating persists, is accompanied by alarming symptoms, or is associated with chronic conditions, seeking guidance from a healthcare professional is imperative. Additionally, if bloating coincides with fever, bloody stool, severe vomiting, or prolonged symptoms, consulting a medical professional is advisable.

Tips for Relieving Constipation

Relieving constipation often involves lifestyle changes and simple interventions. Here are some tips that may help:

Increase Fiber Intake: Consume more fiber-rich foods, such as fruits, vegetables, whole grains, and legumes. Gradually introduce fiber to your diet to avoid bloating or gas. Aim for at least twenty-five to thirty grams of fiber per day.

Stay Hydrated: Drink plenty of water throughout the day to soften stools and aid in digestion. Limit caffeine and alcohol intake, as they can contribute to dehydration.

Regular Physical Activity: Engage in regular exercise to stimulate bowel movements and promote overall digestive health. Even a short daily walk can be beneficial.

Include Probiotics: Consume probiotic-rich foods, like yogurt, or take probiotic supplements to promote a healthy gut microbiome.

Prunes and Fiber-Rich Foods: Prunes (dried plums) are a natural remedy for constipation. They contain both fiber and a natural laxative. Include other fiber-rich foods like bran cereal or oatmeal in your diet.

Limit Processed Foods: Reduce the intake of processed and low-fiber foods, as they can contribute to constipation.

Consider Natural Laxatives: Certain foods, like flaxseeds, chia seeds, and aloe vera, may have natural laxative effects. Be cautious with over-the-counter laxatives and consult a healthcare professional before using them regularly.

Warm Beverages: Warm liquids, such as herbal tea or warm water with lemon, can stimulate bowel movements (Meacham, n.d.).

If constipation persists or becomes a recurring issue, it's essential to consult with a healthcare provider to rule out any underlying conditions and determine an appropriate course of action. They can provide personalized advice based on your health and medical history.

Managing Diarrhea with Proper Hydration and Diet

Consuming bland foods, particularly those included in the BRAT diet (bananas, rice, applesauce, toast), can expedite the resolution of diarrhea and alleviate stomach discomfort.

Here are some tips to manage diarrhea through dietary choices:

Foods to Include in a Bland Diet:

- BRAT diet includes bananas, white rice, applesauce, and white bread toast.

- Additional options: cooked cereals, soda crackers, low-sugar apple juice, boiled potatoes.

BRAT Diet Benefits:

- These foods are bland and low in fiber, aiding in stool firming.

- Accelerates recovery from diarrhea.

- Prevents stomach upset and irritation.

Diet-Diarrhea Connection:
- Diarrhea causes vary, and can include allergies, food poisoning, or chronic conditions like irritable bowel syndrome.

- Long-term digestive conditions can be influenced by your food choices.

- Certain foods can either help restore digestive balance or worsen symptoms during episodes of diarrhea.

Hydration Importance:
- Stay hydrated to replace lost fluids during diarrhea.

- Recommended liquids: water, clear broths (without grease), electrolyte-enhanced water, weak tea.

Post-Recovery Food Introduction:
- Gradually reintroduce foods like scrambled eggs and cooked vegetables as recovery progresses (Seitz, 2023).

Gallstones

Another prominent digestive issue, particularly experienced by women, is the presence of gallstones. When cholesterol gathers inside the gallbladder, it hardens. This can cause pain in the upper-right abdomen or the center of the stomach. Even though the pain typically lasts a few hours, it can be very severe. In most cases, the gallbladder has to be removed through surgery so that the symptoms don't increase. If the surgery is not performed correctly, the person can experience high temperature, chills, nausea and vomiting, accelerated heartbeat, pale-yellow and itchy skin, loss of appetite, and diarrhea.

People who are obese and above the age of forty need to be especially careful with their lifestyle so that they don't suffer from gallstones. To avoid the risk, you must include healthy fats in your diet, such as fish and olive oil, remove processed sugars and fried foods, stay hydrated, and hit the treadmill occasionally.

Celiac Disease / Gluten Intolerance

As we delve further into studying digestive issues, let's discuss gluten intolerance and celiac disease. If you think the two diseases are the same, you are not the only one. It's not uncommon to presume so. In this section, I will help to clear up the differences between the two.

People with gluten intolerance get sick after ingesting gluten (a protein found in grains such as wheat and barley) and endure symptoms such as nausea, feeling tired, and bloated.

On the contrary, celiac disease is an autoimmune disease where the body fights against gluten as if it's a virus, causing inflammation and probable damage to the digestive issues. Gluten intolerance can develop at any time in a person's life—some might even be born with it. Whereas people with Celiac disease have an abnormal gene in their body, along with an innumerable number of certain antibodies that fight gluten. Gluten intolerance is much more frequent, affecting 6 percent of the US population. Conversely, celiac disease affects 1 percent of the US population.

While gluten intolerance and celiac disease have their roots in different bodily systems, they both have similar symptoms. For those who experience either, a shift to gluten-free products, like gluten-free flour, is necessary. Exceptional care needs to be taken to not ingest any gluten so that symptoms don't worsen.

Even though there is no cure for the two diseases, keeping the symptoms at bay is easy: don't consume gluten! Yes, it might seem like an incredulous thought at first that you won't be eating wheat. However, gluten-free wheat and flour are readily available in stores and can be used as substitutes. Using gluten-free flour and substitutes such as oats, cornstarch, and nutmeg may help control symptoms. It certainly does not mean you have to restrict dining out. You can find some fun and easy recipes using gluten-free flour so that your taste buds don't have to compromise. All that's required is a little determination on your part!

Irritable Bowel Syndrome

Another conventional digestive issue is IBS (irritable bowel syndrome), which affects 10-15 percent of the adult population in the US. IBS is a mixture of many symptoms, most commonly constituting bloating, abdominal pain, constipation or diarrhea (or switching between the two), excess gas, and mucus in stool. Most often, the syndrome is found in women anytime from their teens to their late forties. Usually, certain foods and mental stress can trigger the symptoms.

Each person may have a different experience and list of symptoms with their IBS. Nevertheless, I can impart some basic knowledge about the kinds of foods you must eat if you are suffering with IBS. First and foremost, drink plenty of water, limit caffeine, and remove dairy products from your diet (since IBS patients are more prone to lactose intolerance). Also, increase your daily fiber intake. Hopefully, these few changes will help in the management of your IBS.

Rare and Complex Gut Issues

While the digestive issues discussed above are manageable and prove to be non-threatening to life in most cases, the gut has its complications. Sometimes, there can be severe and complex issues as well, which can be difficult to control with lifestyle changes and may require surgery.

Crohn's Disease and Ulcerative Colitis

One of these rare diseases is inflammatory bowel disease (IBD). Crohn's disease and ulcerative colitis also come under IBD. While the former can cause inflammation in any part of the gastrointestinal tract, the latter only occurs in the large intestine. However, both exhibit similar symptoms.

The customary diagnoses for these two diseases are blood tests, stool tests, endoscopies, and bowel imaging and scanning. Even though there is currently no cure for IBD, it can be treated with medication, lifestyle changes, surgery, and complementary and alternative medicine. If the directions are followed thoroughly, someone affected with the disease can live a fully productive life.

Case Study

Natalie, now thirty-four, was diagnosed with Crohn's disease nearly a decade ago and suffers from acute symptoms. Most commonly, she experiences inflammation in her small intestine, which causes her to experience harsh abdominal pain, diarrhea, fluctuation in her body weight, and pain in her joints. Moreover, her entire mood is also affected by her health. She was directed to make certain lifestyle changes, such as maintaining a diet rich in fiber and protein—which helped to give her a lot of energy—adding vitamins as supplements and exercising regularly. Medications, such as steroids, immunosuppressants, and antibiotics, are often used to manage this disease.

Gastroparesis

As we continue talking about chronic gut issues, gastroparesis cannot go unnoticed. The disease was discovered in 1958 by a doctor called Richard Kassander who observed something unusual while examining diabetic patients. He discovered that many of them were experiencing gastrointestinal issues such as nausea, vomiting, bloating, and feeling full quickly, even if their blood sugar levels were acceptable. He was intrigued and decided to investigate further.

Kassander discovered that all these stomach ailments were related to one thing: their stomachs were taking longer than usual to empty after eating. The delay in emptying was generating their suffering (Surtini 2021). This discovery was significant because it was the first time anyone had detected this problem in diabetics. He named it diabetic gastroparesis.

More recently, a study was conducted on a forty-six-year-old man who had been vomiting for five months when he was eventually admitted to Queen Elizabeth Central Hospital. He would vomit at least five times a day and complained of constipation. Apart from being diagnosed with diabetes mellitus 2, there were no other possible causes that were found (Zhang et. al, 2011). After running some tests and observing his symptoms, he was also diagnosed with diabetic gastroparesis.

When specifically related to diabetes, it has been seen to occur when the nerves that control the stomach muscles are destroyed over time because of high blood sugar levels. This causes the stomach to empty abnormally, making the person feel full very soon after starting a meal. They may also experience bloating, abdominal pain, severe nausea and vomiting, loss of appetite, heartburn, fluctuations in blood sugar levels, and constipation.

According to healthcare professionals, to manage this condition, patients should eat smaller and more frequent meals low in fat and fiber content so that they are easy to digest and don't put a strain on their gut. Metoclopramide is often used to treat gastroparesis, as it encourages muscles in the stomach to contract and empty the stomach.

Even though we are still learning about this disease, with the proper treatment, the symptoms can be managed.

Diverticulitis

Moving our discussion from gastroparesis to diverticulitis, we encounter another problematic and painful disease. Some people develop small sacs on the intestinal lining of the colon, known as diverticula. While diverticula are harmless, sometimes they can get inflamed and cause diverticulitis. Symptoms range from severe abdominal pain and high fever to inflammation and changes in bowel movement.

However, the cause of the disease is unknown. While diverticulosis is common, only 4 percent of those with the disease experience inflammation in the diverticula and develop diverticulitis.

Patients with diverticulitis need to avoid nuts, seeds, and popcorn because these become stuck in the diverticula, causing inflammation to occur and flare-up diverticulitis.

Cancer

Just like cancer can affect any part of the body, it can be fatal to the stomach as well. Cells start producing uncontrollably, lining where the stomach meets the esophagus, which is more common in the US, or in the main part of the stomach, which is usually found in other countries.

These cells can start building up, leading to a tumor that can later spread to other body parts, such as the pancreas and liver, if not removed. In the initial stages, symptoms are not felt physically. However, when they do start showing up, the person must visit a healthcare official as soon as possible to be tested. Typical symptoms for cancer are loss of appetite, losing a considerable amount of weight without any apparent reason, weakness and constantly feeling tired, nausea and vomiting, black stool, blood in vomit, feeling bloated, and severe stomach pain.

Despite the fact that there is no particular reason why the genetic mutation occurs that causes cancer, certain common factors have been found in people who have this mutation. It's common in males above sixty-five, whose ethnicity originates in East Asia, South or Central America, or Eastern Europe. If someone has a family history of cancer, they are more prone to the occurrence of genetic mutations. Other risk factors include smoking, having a diet with high salt and fats and low in vegetables and fruits, and suffering with other gastric issues on a regular basis.

To lower the risk of getting stomach or colon cancer, eat a low-salt diet and increase vegetable and fruit intake for nutrition. Quitting smoking is highly suggested as well. In cases where cancer does develop, several procedures can be carried out, such as tumor-removing surgery, chemotherapy, radiation, and immunotherapy. Sometimes they are used in combination with each other for the best results. Stomach cancer is indeed curable if it's diagnosed at an early stage. However, typically it's found when a certain amount of time has passed. So, it's best to stay vigilant by employing the methods suggested here to avoid such a circumstance.

Leaky Gut

Leaky gut syndrome is the starting point of most digestive symptoms and diseases. Our gut is semi-permeable; basically, it allows certain things to pass through, like nutrition, and filters out toxins and bad bacteria. Certain people develop an increased permeability, which allows other toxins to pass through as well. There is no medical diagnosis for the condition, and it has no particular cause behind it.

However, it has been found that autoimmune diseases that affect the digestive system cause a leaky gut. In other cases, it was found that certain patients had leaky gut before they were diagnosed with these diseases. It isn't known whether it is the cause of a disease, just another symptom, or if it can be classified as a disease in itself. Regardless, awareness is increasing that leaky gut syndrome is a foundational problem and that it is related to various disease processes.

So, what happens when you have a leaky gut?

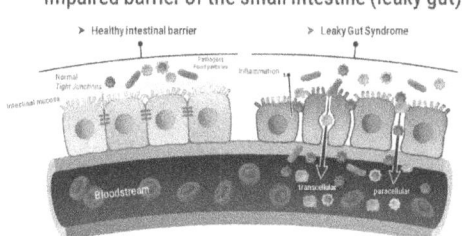

(Image from Alcat-europe – Leaky gut syndrome)

Effects of Leaky Gut

At this point, we have established that an unhappy gut is an unhappy you. The following points highlight how leaky gut syndrome affects the whole digestive system and, in turn, affects your overall health.

- Leaky gut can cause inflammation, which causes your immune system to weaken. It begins to react to every little microbiome in the body, even good ones, which then cause diseases such as IBDs and arthritis.

- The continual flooding of toxins and bad microbes into the bloodstream causes gut dysbiosis. This is where the bad microbiome increases, creating an imbalance in the gut.

- Additionally, your gut has a lot of bacteria that are responsible for digesting lactose, gluten, and other foods. With a leaky gut, they all flow out, and the bigger molecules of food, like proteins, cannot be digested fully, causing food intolerance.

- The improper in-and-out flow of nutrients through the bloodstream can also cause nutrient malabsorption, for example, anemia. Moreover, as we've previously seen, gut health hugely impacts your mental health, as an imbalanced gut may disrupt the gut-brain axis, leading to the potential of anxiety and depression.

Gut Check!

The Belly Blueprint Quiz
- How is your daily fruit intake?

1. Fruit? What's that?

2. I eat fruit every few days.

3. I eat fruit daily.

4. I eat loads of fruit daily!

- How many portions of vegetables do you consume daily?

1. I don't eat vegetables at all.

2. I try to eat at least one serving of vegetables a day.

3. I usually eat two servings of vegetables a day.

4. My daily diet is full of tasty vegetables!

- Do you stay hydrated throughout the day?

1. I barely drink any water.

2. I drink 0.5 liters of water a day.

3. I drink about 0.5- 1 liter of water a day.

4. I drink 2 or more liters of water a day.

- How much caffeine do you consume per day? (Includes coffee, tea, caffeinated soft drinks, energy drinks, etc.)

1. I barely drink caffeinated drinks.

2. About 1-2 cups a day.

3. 3 cups a day.

4. 4 or more cups a day.

- How many probiotic foods (yogurt, kefir, etc.) do you eat on a weekly basis?

1. Barely any.

2. 1 serving weekly.

3. About 2-3 servings weekly.

4. More than 3 servings weekly.

- Does your daily diet contain nuts, seeds, or beans?

1. I don't usually have those.

2. About 1-2 servings.

3. 3 servings.

4. More than 4 servings.

- Would you describe your diet as a healthy diet?

1. I eat whatever is convenient, whether it's healthy or not.

2. I try to make my meals as healthy as possible.

3. They are somewhat healthy with a few exceptions at times.

4. It's strictly healthy. I barely eat any extra carbs or fats.

- How many hours do you give yourself after dinner before you go to sleep?

1. I sleep immediately.

2. 1-2 hours.

3. 2-3 hours.

4. 4 or more hours.

- How frequent are your bowel movements?

1. I go once a day, and sometimes not even daily.

2. It's usually once a day.

3. It's twice a day on average.

4. At least three times a day.

- How's your mental state throughout the week?

1. I am fairly unhappy.

2. I am mostly neutral.

3. I feel happy.

- How many hours of sleep do you get every night?

1. I get 5 or less hours of sleep.

2. I sleep 5-7 hours a day.

3. I sleep 7-8 hours a day.

4. I sleep more than 10 hours.

- How often do you exercise for at least thirty minutes to the point that you are short of breath?

1. Sometimes once a week, sometimes I don't at all.

2. About 1-2 times a week.

3. 3-4 times a week.

4. Every. Single. Day. I love working out!

- How often are you bothered by gut discomfort?

1. Less than once a month.

2. About 1 to 3 times a month.

3. Every week.

4. 3 or more times a week.

- Do you take medication or any drugs?

1. Yes.

2. No.

- Do you have health conditions, such as diabetes or blood pressure, running in your family?

1. Yes.

2. No.

I hope you learned something new about yourself in this quiz. You may have discovered that you have a fairly healthy gut, but if, unfortunately, your gut is not healthy and you scored low numbers on this quiz, you need to prioritize yourself and your health more.

What if I told you that what happens in your stomach also directly affects your mood? What if I told you that certain foods can help elevate your mood and aid in removing depression? Incredulous, right? The next chapter will show us how the gut relates to our brain and emotions. It might help you during the times you feel low.

Chapter Three

The Gut-Brain Connection

"*Recent studies suggest that in close interactions with its resident microbes, the gut can influence our basic emotions, our pain sensitivity, and our social interactions, and even guide many of our decisions—and not just those about our food preferences and meal sizes.*"
- Emeran Mayer

The gut-brain connection is remarkable. As communication is bidirectional, it not only serves the digestive system but is also significant in our mental well-being. It's important to understand this connection if you plan to improve your physical and mental health.

Exploring the Gut-Brain Axis

Have you ever been in a situation where you did not logically know what to do, but in the end, you decided to go with your gut? Have you ever experienced butterflies in your stomach when you are nervous about talking to someone you like?

If so, then you already know that our gut and mind are intricately linked with each other. They pass information between each other, discussing all sorts of matters— practical, physical, and emotional—just like best friends do! This connection between your gut and brain is called the gut-brain axis.

In its bidirectional communication, the nerves send information from the gut to the central nervous system and then back from the central nervous system to the gut. The information exchanged can be related to your hunger, food preferences, food intolerances, muscle movements, digestion, metabolism, mood, stress levels, pain sensitivity, cognitive functions, and immunity.

The response that you feel with every exchange of information can vary from fast and potent to gentle and pleasurable. If you get food poisoning and urgently have the need to go to the washroom to empty your bowels, you will experience a fast and potent exchange of information. On the other hand, if you're having a warm cup of hot chocolate on a winter evening, the effect will be gentle and pleasing.

According to clinical evidence, the number of microbes in the gut directly affects the gut-brain axis. Many disorders, such as anxiety, depression, and autism have been shown to have a link with disturbances in the gut. In addition, your diet directly affects your gut, and eventually your cognition. Several studies have proven a link between depression and inflamed cytokines (proteins that help control inflammation in the body). Hence why, in severe depression, patients are given anti-inflammatory drugs, such as COX-2 inhibitors.

In 2017, an experiment was conducted on a sample of forty people with depression. They were asked to take the Beck Depression Inventory test, and their initial responses were recorded. They were then given probiotics (L acidophilus, L casei, and Bifidobacterium bifidum) for eight weeks before taking the Beck Depression Inventory test again.

Their responses on the test improved, further proving that having a healthier gut has a significant impact on our mental health (Appleton, 2018).

Through research, we have come to understand that the gut microbiome produces several neurotransmitters that affect mood and cognition. A balanced microbiome community helps keep mood stable and happy, while an imbalance in microbes can cause the inhibition of adequate neurotransmitters. This can lead to an increase in stress levels, and in severe cases, even cause anxiety and depression.

An imbalanced microbiome can also cause internal inflammation, which again lowers the production of required neurotransmitters, leading the person back to an imbalanced microbiome and at an increased risk for lower mood.

Now, we all know the common hormones (neurotransmitters) that determine your happy mood: serotonin and dopamine. Initially, we thought that these hormones were produced in the brain only. However, we now know that many of these are also produced in the gut. For this reason, the gut is also known as the 'second brain.'

Serotonin

Serotonin is a mood-balancing hormone that helps stabilize emotions. Not only does it keep anxiety at bay, but it also helps with digestion, healing wounds, keeping your bowel movements active and functioning normally, and maintaining your bone density. It also activates mucus and fluid secretion inside the digestive system for absorption in the intestine. Serotonin controls nerve receptors as well, which means that it tells you when you feel bloated or are in pain.

The body deals efficiently with serotonin, as any excess is converted to melatonin to help you sleep. Lack of serotonin can be responsible for depression, anxiety, chronic pain, insomnia, and memory issues.

Production and Availability of Serotonin

We now know that 95 percent of serotonin is produced in the gut, while the remaining 5 percent is produced in the brain. Serotonin can only be produced when the gut has the required nutrients to produce it. Nutrients such as vitamin C, vitamin B9, zinc, and omega-3 are essential for the production of serotonin. It really can't be overstated how vital of a role nutrition plays in mental health.

Neurotransmitter Hormones

Dopamine is a neurotransmitter that is necessary for maintaining focus, awareness, productivity, and reproductivity. A lack of dopamine can cause anxiety, an inability to focus, muscle stiffness, and indigestion. 50 percent of dopamine production is carried out in the gut, further reinforcing the importance of the gut-brain axis.

GABA (the major neurotransmitter in the spinal cord that stimulates the production of insulin) is produced in the pancreas, which, if you remember, is also part of the digestive system. GABA reduces stress and anxiety, allowing for relaxation. A lack of it is known to increase the risk of depression, insomnia, and a lack of concentration.

Other neurotransmitter hormones, like norepinephrine (the body's stress response hormone), are also produced in the gut. If your body experiences too much stress and releases a lot of norepinephrine, the excess goes into the gut and weakens the immune system.

Gut-Nourishing Foods

I am often asked, "How can I be happier?" Though there is no one treatment for it, and several mental disorders require you to visit a professional for proper treatment, it is still worth trying a few methods to elevate your mood. In the end, fighting depression requires your own will and steadfastness. The research discussed in this chapter has shown that the gut is very much responsible for our mental health, so the immediate course of action is to improve your routine and remain committed to it, starting with food.

Several of my patients battle with anxiety and mood swings, especially in the presence of various digestive issues. I tell them one thing—your diet determines almost everything, from your health to your mood.

Lisa, aged forty-three, is a mother of two and a high school teacher. For a few months, she was experiencing frequent mood swings and irritability. She felt that sometimes she became passive-aggressive as well with her kids or students. Her work requires her to stay focused and plan lectures accordingly, but she felt she was unable to do her job well because she lacked focus.

She realized that because of her tiring routine, she could not make the time to prepare food herself, which meant eating processed food. After careful discussion, I gave her a simple diet plan that did not require lengthy processes of cooking and suggested she go for a brisk walk for thirty minutes at least four days a week. Five months after her initial check-up, she admitted to feeling much lighter, happier, and focused on her life.

So, what exactly should we be eating to improve our mood?

Foods That Promote Gut Health

As mentioned before, our bodies need prebiotics and probiotics to have a healthier gut. Prebiotics help digestion, control blood sugar levels, and aid in nutrient absorption. Scientists in San Jose University, Boston, Massachusetts, have declared these five foods to be the best sources for prebiotics: garlic, leeks, onions, dandelion greens, and Jerusalem artichokes. These foods contain about 100-240 milligrams of prebiotics in one gram. On average, an adult human should eat five grams of prebiotics a day.

Nutrient-Rich Foods

Vitamin C is found in citrus fruits like oranges and lemons. It enables the body to process carbohydrates, fats, and proteins. Vitamin C

UNDERSTANDING LEAKY GUT & HORMONES... 53

is also an important component in the making of neurotransmitters, such as serotonin, dopamine, and norepinephrine—the hormones that keep depression at a far distance.

In 2018, a study conducted on 139 young men found that those with a good amount of vitamin C in their blood showed the lowest signs of depression (Plevin 2020). For premenstrual depression, vitamin B6 is quite effective. Just like with vitamin C, our bodies require vitamin B6 to produce neurotransmitters.

Additionally, folate—a form of vitamin B9—helps create more cells and DNA, as well as encouraging the production of serotonin, eventually enhancing mood. Another nutrient, magnesium, found in tofu and whole grains, keeps a check on hormonal balance.

And, according to research, it has been found that people with heavy depression often have extremely low zinc levels. Zinc supplements can, therefore, be very therapeutic for people struggling with severe depression.

Last, but not least, since our brain is 60 percent fat, it requires good fats to function well. Omega-3 has been seen to have a significant impact on brain function, reducing the risk of depression in children and adults. The best sources of omega-3 foods are chia seeds, flax seeds, and fish—particularly wild salmon, herring, and sardines. These are low in mercury and high in omega-3. Walnuts also contain a lot of omega-3, as well as helping to lower blood pressure by keeping arteries clean.

To ensure you maintain optimal brain power, eat a good amount of leafy vegetables daily, such as lettuce, spinach, and broccoli. Berries have also been shown to help memory, as proven by researchers at Harvard's Brigham and Women's Hospital (Harvard 2021).

Gut-Friendly Lifestyle Practices for Emotional Balance

Maintaining a healthy gut to achieve good mental health will take time, commitment, and effort. In addition to eating the right foods, including prebiotics, probiotics, and other nutrients, you also need to exercise or do some form of physical workout to activate your gut. You can choose whatever you're comfortable with and enjoy doing, whether walking, jogging, hitting the gym, or even dancing! All you need is 150 minutes a week to sweat. This can help increase the good bacteria in your body by as much as 40 percent.

Besides eating healthily and exercising, try to avoid antibiotics as much as possible. The use of excessive antibiotics can remove the good bacteria as well as the bad from your gut, which can lower your immunity in the long run. Often small issues can be fixed by simple home remedies. If an antibiotic is necessary, take a probiotic at the same time to minimize the assault on your good bacteria.

Gut Health Practices for Enhancing Emotional Resilience and Coping Mechanisms

The most important aspect in keeping your mind healthy is keeping stress low. Although, this is often easier said than done. My immediate response to being stressed used to be binge eating dessert and comfort food. However, I have changed this over the years, and now I try to help other people change their unhealthy reactions to stress, too. You *can* deal with stress using healthy coping mechanisms.

Relaxation Techniques

Start with taking some deep breaths to help your body relax and to regulate your nervous system, calming the fight-or-flight response.

I find the best way to de-stress during a situation is to immediately write about how I'm feeling. I suggest you keep a small journal in your bag, and whenever you feel your emotions are becoming overwhelming, take five minutes and write about it.

Another way to eliminate stressful thoughts about a situation is to think positively, finding the good in a bad situation. Here's an example: you worked really hard for a promotion that was long due, but you didn't get it. This situation can be very demotivating. But it's important to remember that it is not a representation of your skill and hard work. Perhaps you will be rewarded in some other way.

Another idea is to dress up and socialize with your friends; laughing and talking with them can provide you with a good temporary distraction from your stress. They also might have a new perspective on your situation, which could be helpful.

Relaxation or meditation techniques are especially helpful. They can help you pinpoint your emotions and remove the negative energy from within you. One such methodology is the autogenic technique. In this, you use imagery to visualize a peaceful moment or repeat words or phrases that make you feel calm. Then, you focus on your body sensations, being mindful of how each body part reacts, and also noticing your breathing.

The progressive muscle relaxation technique promotes relaxation, too, but utilizes a different method than the autogenic technique. In this, you tense your muscles intentionally and then loosen them to determine the difference between tense muscles because of stress and muscles in a state of relaxation. You start by sitting in a quiet room, devoid of any distractions. You then tense and relax the muscles in your neck for a minute. Next, you work your way down to your shoulders, then the abdomen, your legs, and finally your toes. This technique is especially helpful in making you more aware of your body.

The third technique, visualization, is similar to the autogenic technique. You sit in a quiet room as relaxed as possible with your shoulders dropped. You may want to close your eyes. Think of a scene that makes you happy and relaxed. For example, sitting by the river where you can hear the gushing sound of the flowing water. Try adding as many elements as you can and want, such as lighting, sunlight, the wind, subjects, and people. Take deep breaths in and out and focus on relaxing your muscles.

Other relaxation techniques include massage, yoga, music therapy, aromatherapy, and hydrotherapy. If you practice these techniques regularly, they can help elevate your mood.

You can also plan a longer time of relaxation—your own self-care week! Here are some ideas for how that could look. Choose to do a thirty-minute simple yoga when you wake up and before breakfast. Yoga helps you stretch your body, strengthen your muscles, and wake up your senses. Then, make an informed choice on the kind of breakfast you want, ensuring it contains enough probiotics and prebiotics. In the evening, go for a thirty-minute brisk walk in nature, and allow yourself to breathe fresh air. If you have a dog, take it out for a run. Your lunch and dinner should include vegetables and fruits, which give you healthy nutrients. Make sure you leave three hours in between your dinner and sleeping time.

On the weekend, take time out for your friends and socialize with them. In addition to that, find some personal 'me' time for yourself, too, doing things that you enjoy. Perhaps you enjoy going out shopping or you like to spread paint on a canvas and create art. Whatever you do, have at least one day to yourself in a week when you can destress yourself. Because the secret to living a happy life is not taking on stress—and a healthy gut!

The next chapter discusses in detail what specific nutrients the organs need to perform best so that you may incorporate them into your daily diet. It will also talk about why it's important to eat mindfully and how it affects your digestion and mood. So, let's read on.

CHAPTER FOUR

Nourishing Your Digestive System

> *"The road to good health is paved with good intestines."*
> - Sherry A. Rogers

Welcome to chapter 4, where we're delving into the fascinating world of your digestive system. In the next few pages, we'll uncover the secrets of maintaining a healthy gut.

Here's the plan: this chapter is all about your gut. The goal? To provide you with the essential tools to develop a diet and lifestyle that perfectly aligns with your digestive system. We're not just focusing on what's on your plate; we're exploring a holistic approach to nurturing your gut.

Are you ready to unlock the wonders of nourishment? Let's embark on this journey together as we explore the basic methods for healing your gut through diet and lifestyle choices. Get ready for a personalized and transformative experience!

Balanced Eating for Gut Health

Have you ever contemplated how to maintain a balanced diet for your overall well-being, including the health of your gut? But you didn't know where to start, or perhaps you started and got discouraged with how overwhelming it felt? This section will give you tools and tips to get started and stay on track. Let's navigate through it together.

Sustaining good health and feeling your best heavily relies on maintaining a healthy, balanced diet. While certain groups, such as athletes, might need additional support through protein supplements, most individuals can adequately meet their nutritional needs by embracing a diverse range of foods.

A balanced diet not only fuels your body for effective function but is also instrumental in supporting gut health. Optimal gut function is achieved by consuming a variety of foods, while minimizing the intake of salt, sugars, and saturated fats.

Neglecting a balanced diet can lead to declining nutrient levels, exposing a significant portion of the population to the risk of vitamin deficiencies. Consequences may include problems with digestion, anemia, and skin issues.

Here, we will explore the essentials of a balanced diet, its significance, and practical tips for meeting your nutritional needs daily, with a special focus on how it contributes to maintaining a healthy gut.

Understanding a Balanced Diet

A balanced diet ideally encompasses five food groups, as emphasized by Isabel Maples, a registered dietitian. Each group contributes essential nutrients, such as vitamins, minerals, fiber, and calories. The Dietary Guidelines from the U.S. Department of Agriculture recommend nutrient-dense foods, placing importance on fruits, vegetables, whole grains, dairy, protein foods, and oils (Renton, 2022). These guidelines also stress the importance of limiting added sugars, saturated fats, sodium, and alcohol.

Variety is crucial, particularly concerning the consumption of fruits and vegetables, which also play a key role in promoting a healthy gut. Nutritionist Lamorna Hollingsworth advises aiming for at least five portions a day, regardless of whether they are fresh, frozen, canned, or dried (Renton 2022).

Practical Tips for Maintaining a Balanced Diet Every Day

While a healthy diet includes all necessary nutrients and food groups, maintaining balance is crucial. The plate method, endorsed by Maples, divides your plate into portions for fruits and vegetables, grains, and protein, with dairy on the side. Individualized needs can be assessed using the USDA's MyPlate Plan.

Hollingsworth emphasizes viewing food on a spectrum to avoid labeling it as good or bad. This approach not only promotes overall balance but also fosters gut health, by encouraging the consumption of a variety of foods that nourish the microbiome.

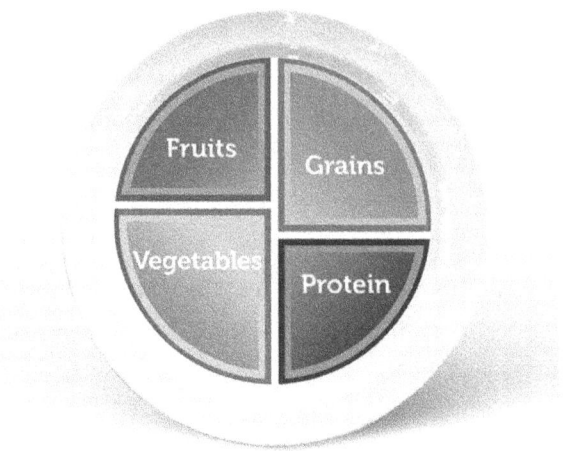

(Image from choosemyplate.gov)

The Power of Probiotics and Prebiotics

As we talked about in Chapter 1, prebiotics are non-digestible fibers that become a feast for the superheroes in your gut: beneficial bacteria. They are the backbone of a healthy gut microbiome, responsible for digestion, immune system harmony, and even mental well-being.

In my journey to better gut health, I found that by incorporating prebiotic-rich foods like chicory root, Jerusalem artichoke, garlic, onions, and bananas into my diet, I witnessed a happier gut, less inflammation, and a newfound energy. It has been truly transformative.

I also started adding more fruits and vegetables to my meals, especially those with complex carbohydrates. These carbs, like fiber and resistant starch, don't get digested by my body. Instead, they become a banquet for bacteria and other microbe rockstars. And when they reach the colon, it's like a celebration. Fermentation occurs, and short-chain fatty acids join the party, bringing a bunch of health perks, such as boosting the immune system, feeling satisfied, and better nutrient absorption. It's like a gut fiesta!

Probiotic-Rich Foods to Add to Your Diet

Have you ever wondered where to find these beneficial bacteria? Well, here's a list of seventeen foods that I personally turn to for their rich probiotic content.

1. Kefir: A fermented dairy product similar to yogurt, originating from Russia and Turkey over 3,000 years ago, known for its slightly acidic and tart flavor.

2. Sauerkraut: A German favorite, made from fermented cabbage and other probiotic vegetables, it's high in organic acids which support the growth of good bacteria.

3. Kombucha: An effervescent fermentation of black tea with primary health benefits including digestive support, increased energy, and liver detoxification.

4. Coconut Kefir: Fermented from the juice of young coconuts with kefir grains, it offers a tropical twist along with several strains of beneficial probiotics.

5. Natto: A Japanese dish of fermented soybeans containing the powerful probiotic Bacillus subtilis, known for boosting the immune system and supporting cardiovascular health.

6. Yogurt: A popular probiotic food made from the milk of cows, goats, or sheep. It does have variations in quality, so opt for organic, grass-fed varieties.

7. Kvass: A traditional Eastern European fermented beverage, historically made from rye or barley, now created using probiotic fruits, beets, and other root vegetables.

8. Raw Cheese: High in probiotics, including thermophillus, bifidus, bulgaricus, and acidophilus. Choose raw and unpasteurized options for maximum benefits.

9. Apple Cider Vinegar: Known for controlling blood pressure, reducing cholesterol, and aiding in weight loss, it can also contribute to your probiotic intake.

10. Salted Gherkin Pickles: A lesser-known source of probiotics. Choose smaller, organic producers for the best health benefits.

11. Brine-Cured Olives: An excellent probiotic source when brine-cured. Select organic and smaller brands to ensure maximum probiotic content.

12. Tempeh: A fermented soybean product from Indonesia, it's versatile and rich in probiotics, suitable for various culinary uses.

13. Miso: A traditional Japanese spice created by fermenting soybean, barley, or brown rice with koji, known for its use in miso soup and macrobiotic cooking.

14. Traditional Buttermilk: A fermented drink made from the liquid left after churning butter, best when containing live cultures for probiotic benefits.

15. Water Kefir: A fizzy, fermented beverage made by adding

UNDERSTANDING LEAKY GUT & HORMONES... 63

grains to sugar water, offering a natural, vegan probiotic option with customizable flavors.

16. Raw Milk: High in probiotics, particularly when raw and unpasteurized, making it a superior choice compared to pasteurized options.

Kimchi: The Korean counterpart to sauerkraut. A flavorful mix of fermented vegetables that adds a probiotic boost to your meals.

More Incredible Foods for Gut Health

Now, let's talk about other delicious foods your gut will love. Based on personal experiences and lots of research, here are my recommendations:

- Bananas: Especially the green ones. They're like magic for your gut, and I can vouch for it!

- Artichokes, Broccoli, and Green Peas: Vegetables that are not just good for your taste buds but also pack a punch of fibers and antioxidants for a happy gut.

- Whole Grains: Think oats, brown rice, and whole grain bread. They're like a feast for your gut bacteria fan club.

- Seafood With Omega-3 Fatty Acids: Fish like salmon and mackerel are full of anti-inflammatory powers, promoting gut happiness.

- Fermented Foods: Yogurt, sauerkraut, kimchi, and kombucha are the cool kids with prebiotics that throw the best gut parties.

- Foods with Polyphenols: Dark chocolate, green tea, and red wine—these treats are not just for your taste buds but also a boost for your gut bacteria.

- Almonds: They're not just snacks; they're gut-loving heroes packed with fiber and beneficial fatty acids.

- Ginger: The spicy superhero aiding digestion is a must-have for a happy gut.

- Lean Proteins: Chicken, turkey, eggs, and tofu are not just delicious but also inflammation fighters and gut-lining repair experts. Low-Fructose Fruits: Strawberries, oranges, and blueberries. These fruity delights are gentle on digestion and won't cause a ruckus.

What is the best way to incorporate these into your daily routine? Simple swaps and creative recipes are the key. Substitute soda for kombucha, regular yogurt for the probiotic kind, and experiment with tempeh or sauerkraut for added flavor. Get creative, try new things, and let these probiotic-rich foods enhance your health.

Hydration and its Impact on Digestion

Have you ever thought about the connection between staying hydrated and keeping your gut healthy? We have already talked about how our diet impacts gut health, but let's explore the role that hydration plays in this digestive process.

Water is more than just a drink to quench your thirst; it's a crucial player in various bodily functions, from digestion and nutrient absorption to waste elimination and temperature regulation. Dehydration can actually worsen digestive symptoms, such as constipation and bloating.

So, how does hydration affect gut health? Picture water as the guiding force that helps food move through your digestive tract. It's like the extra push that ensures you have regular bathroom trips. If you're dealing with constipation, increasing your water intake might be the solution.

Here's an interesting fact: Fiber, the superhero nutrient for gut health, needs water as its sidekick. Without enough fluid, too much fiber can lead to discomfort and constipation. Your body might pull extra fluid from the large intestine, making stools hard to pass—a situation you do not want to find yourself in.

Did you know that constipation is the most common cause of bloating? When someone comes to me expressing concerns about bloating, the first thing I check is whether they're dealing with constipation.

Now, let's talk about the practical aspect: How much water do you need? Well, it varies depending on factors like metabolism, environment, and physical activity. As a rough guide, Dietitians of Canada suggest around 2.2 liters (nine cups) for women and 3 liters (twelve cups) for men. Keep in mind that this is a general figure; your unique needs might differ. The more general recommendation is eight cups a day.

Feeling overwhelmed by those water goals? Don't worry! Solid foods contribute about 20 percent of your total water intake. Fruits and veggies, in particular, are packed with water.

For those who find it challenging to drink enough water to take care of the other 80 percent, fear not! There are strategies that can help. Sipping through a straw has been shown to increase water intake. Adding a dash of flavor with mint, citrus, or berries can make hydration more enjoyable. And consider sparkling water since it's a bubbly twist to your plain H2O. To make things easier, carry a water bottle everywhere: in your car, at your desk, you name it.

So, there you have it. A little hydration equals a happy gut. Keep sipping and let your digestive system thank you. Here's to a hydrated and healthy you!

Mindful Eating Practices for Better Digestion

We've all experienced that familiar belly swell after a meal we couldn't resist (the regret of overindulging). It's like a post-feast adventure with buttons popping and cramps setting in. That literal *gut feeling* demands our attention.

Our gut, functioning as the Chief Operating Officer (COO) of our body, holds significant influence. Ever heard of the Enteric Nervous System (ENS)? It's like a hidden brain in our digestive system, impacting our health, mood, and thoughts. Some of us heed its warnings and steer clear of problematic foods, while others persist until resistance builds.

The twist in the tale is this: what you feed your gut matters most. Your food choices dictate your digestive health. The COO sends messages to the brain (the Chief Executive Officer or CEO), triggering various responses. Consume unhealthy foods, and you might find yourself dealing with adult acne, joint pain, or even a canvas of rashes. All because the COO disapproves.

If we're all about becoming healthier, it's time to keep the COO content. A balanced diet, hydration, daily exercise, and quality sleep are the keys to a happy COO. Cut back on culprits like dairy, processed meats, and refined sugars, and witness your gut thriving.

Maintaining a food diary can help you to identify trigger foods—those that leave you feeling low, ones that bring on that unwelcome belly swell, or leave you experiencing other uncomfortable digestive issues. Your gut will thank you for becoming more mindful.

Mindful Eating and its Impact on Digestion

When we embrace mindful eating, we're not just having a meal; we're unlocking a treasure trove of benefits for our overall well-being. By being fully present during our eating experiences, we turbocharge our body's ability to absorb those essential nutrients, creating a healthier digestive haven.

Mindful eating is like a nutrient-absorption superhero. Why? Well, when we're all in on the present moment, our senses kick into high gear and better digestion and absorption follow suit. It's like a nutrient party where we get VIP treatment.

But wait, there's more. Mindful eating isn't just about savoring each bite (though that's pretty awesome); it's a stressbuster, too. Stress messes with nutrient absorption and our gut buddies. However, when we're Zen-like during meals, stress takes a backseat, paving the way for optimal digestion and a thriving gut environment.

A quick tip: Make mindful eating a lifestyle, not just a temporary fling. Despite life's distractions, dedicating yourself to this practice pays off big time. Think about your digestive system doing a happy dance at the improved nutrient absorption as you chew slowly and focus on the sensory delight of eating.

But that's not all, mindful eating is your body's BFF when it comes to hunger signals. No more mindless snacking or overeating. Plus, it's your detective tool to uncover any food triggers or intolerances. Pro tip: Throw in some deep breaths before meals. It's a digestion booster.

Incorporating Mindfulness into Mealtimes

Here are six core tips for mindful eating exercises:

- Use all your senses: Appreciate flavors, colors, and textures.

- Eat slowly: Enjoy each bite, focusing on taste and recognizing fullness.

- No distractions: Put away gadgets and give your meal your

full attention.

- Be thankful: Express gratitude for your food's source.

- Listen to your body: Pay attention to hunger and fullness cues.

- Understand emotional eating: Recognize triggers for overeating.

Mindful eating isn't a temporary fix; it's a lifestyle change. Consistency is key for lasting improvements in nutrient absorption and digestive well-being. Take it one bite at a time—little mindful eating adventures for lasting changes in digestive health. If you plan ahead, you can include a variety of healthy options in meals, bringing an interesting variety to your diet.

Mindful eating also encourages other positive changes in everyday life. Because it boosts awareness, encourages mindful choices, and focuses on a satisfying experience, this game-changer for digestive health and your relationship with food will also ripple out in other areas.

Now, let's address the challenges of mindful eating. It takes focus, discipline, and resisting unhealthy temptations. Strategies like planning meals, seeking healthier options, and creating dedicated meal spaces can help. Overcoming distractions and societal pressures means communicating your needs and prioritizing digestive health.

Importance of Chewing Food Properly

Have you ever wondered why our grandparents insisted on chewing food slowly? Well, it's not just an old saying—there's some real wisdom there.

Imagine this: you're digging into a tasty meal, and time is not on your side! We've all been there. But here's the catch: When you scarf down your food like there's a race on, it's like sending a jumbled puzzle to your stomach. Conversely, chewing your food thoroughly is like handing your stomach a set of instructions to solving the puzzle.

I used to be the queen of fast food, always in a hurry. But then, I started getting unwelcome visits from indigestion. I decided to pump the brakes and relish every bite, eliminating the discomfort I felt from speed eating.

When you chew your food well, you're essentially turning it into bite-sized pieces. This not only makes your stomach's job easier but also signals to your body that a feast is on the horizon. Your gut is a fan of mindfulness. It's not just about chewing; it's about being in the moment. When you're conscious of what's going into your mouth, your body responds with a nod of appreciation.

So, the next time you're at the dinner table, put away that phone, take a moment, and chew like it's your first taste. Your gut will send you a thank-you note, and you'll be on your way to a digestive masterpiece.

The Do's and Don'ts of a Gut-Healthy Diet

Ever wondered about inflammation? If you've had a cut, bruise, or throat infection, you've probably felt the signs—redness, swelling, pain, and heat. This is acute inflammation, your body's response to illness or injury, and it usually resolves on its own.

Yet, there's another player: systemic inflammation. It affects the entire body and can last too long. Chronic inflammation is linked to serious diseases like obesity, diabetes, heart disease, and certain cancers. Surprisingly, what you eat can fuel inflammation. Red meat, processed snacks, and sugary drinks all encourage inflammation.

Cooking matters, too. Choose baking, steaming, or a quick stir-fry, since deep frying can stir up trouble. In addition to this, label reading is your weapon against inflammation. Sneaky sugars and trans fats hide in processed foods. If it says, "partially hydrogenated oils," steer clear.

So, what are some anti-inflammatory foods? Think omega-3 fatty acids in fish, vitamin C in fruits and veggies, and polyphenols in coffee, tea, and dark chocolate. And don't forget the gut-friendly squad that we discussed earlier: probiotics and prebiotics in fermented foods and fiber-rich treats.

If you are looking for an MVP diet against inflammation, the Mediterranean diet is your go-to playbook. It's all about omega-3s, vitamin C, polyphenols, and fiber-rich goodness.

Ready to make a change? Start small. Swap out inflammatory culprits for healthier alternatives. Like trading charcuterie for veggie slices with hummus or opting for grilled eggplant instead of a burger. It may seem like a challenge, but these tweaks can turn into habits that kick inflammation to the curb.

Remember, no single food is the hero against inflammation, but crafting a wholesome diet is your superpower. It's not just about reducing risk; it's about transforming your health, one mindful meal at a time.

Strategies to Curb Sugar Cravings and Support Gut Health

Let's talk about overcoming sugar cravings and supporting our gut health. It's a real struggle, and I've been there, grabbing for that sugary fix like it's the solution to everything. But you know what? There are ways to beat those cravings and give our gut some love.

First, let's consider the gut microbiota—those little warriors inside your belly. They play a big role in your cravings and food choices. Personally, I have found that adding more fiber-rich foods to my diet makes a difference. Foods like fruits, veggies, and whole grains have become my allies in this battle.

Now, tackling sugar cravings isn't just about willpower; it's a biochemical challenge. When that sweet tooth kicked in, I started choosing natural sweeteners like honey or maple syrup. These small changes had a significant impact. I also noticed that balancing my meals with protein, healthy fats, and fiber-rich foods helped tone down the intensity of my cravings.

Don't underestimate the power of hydration. I began drinking more water, and surprisingly, my cravings became mere whispers instead of loud demands. Water helped me feel full and satisfied the need to snack on something sweet or salty.

I also embraced mindfulness as a new hobby. When a craving hit, I took a moment to breathe, acknowledged the craving without judgment, and questioned whether I was genuinely hungry or just bored. More often than not, it turned out I was just bored.

Finally, I made sure to have healthy snacks on hand. When the sweet tooth struck, having a stash of nuts, Greek yogurt, or dark chocolate (in moderation) saved me from succumbing to sugary temptations.

To all my fellow sugar warriors, it's not about bidding farewell to sweets forever. It's about finding balance, making mindful choices, and letting your gut be your guide. Trust me, your body will thank you, and those sugar cravings will become a thing of the past.

How to Create and Stick with a New Eating Plan

Healthy eating: it's not just about looking good; it's about feeling good and dodging those nasty diseases. An unhealthy diet? Well, that's the express lane to problems like obesity, heart disease, type 2 diabetes, and even certain cancers.

Now, I get it. Dieting is a beast, but trust me, it's a daily investment in yourself that pays off big time. A healthy diet is only partially about shedding pounds. More importantly, it's about boosting your life expectancy, keeping your immune system in top form, lifting your mood, and ramping up your energy levels so you can conquer your day.

But let's talk about the hurdles. Do you feel like you're stuck in an 'all-or-nothing' loop? One where a tiny slip-up feels like a colossal failure? I've been there, and I want to assure you that it's okay not to be perfect. It's normal to struggle with body image but obsessing over how you look can mess with your healthy eating groove. It's about progress, not perfection.

Stress. Oh boy, stress eating is a thing. I've been there, too. Mindless munching when the world feels heavy. Take a breath; it happens to the best of us. And depression? It's no joke. Poor eating habits can be a sign. If you're battling more than just diet demons and feeling hopeless, chat with your healthcare provider. They've got your back!

So, if any of these hurdles hit close to home, don't rush into a diet plan. Pause and figure out what's holding you back, and then dive in.

Now, let's move on to talking about sticking to your diet plan and actually reaching those goals. I've got a few tips that worked wonders for me:

Keep it Real: Set achievable and realistic goals. Don't go for extreme calorie cuts or expect to lose a ton of weight in a short time. It's not healthy or sustainable.

Start Small: Take it easy at the beginning. Instead of banning entire food groups, try setting small goals like treating yourself once a week. Going all-in can make it tough to bounce back after the occasional sweet indulgence.

Prep like a Pro: Spend some time each week prepping meals, especially the ones you love. It makes it way easier to choose a home-cooked meal over hitting the drive-through.

Snack Smart: Keep healthy snacks around, whether you're at the office or at home. Frozen grapes or a bit of dark chocolate beat the vending machine any day. Swap out junk for snacks like parmesan crisps or light white cheddar popcorn, which are just as satisfying without the guilt.

Love Your Plan: If your diet is making you miserable, it's not the right one. Find a plan you enjoy like counting macros, where you can still savor your favorite foods in moderation. Talk to your healthcare provider for guidance and maybe some extra tips.

Remember, dieting doesn't have to be a struggle. It's about getting healthier, not just thinner. Slow and steady wins the race. If you need extra support, consider consulting a trained dietitian.

Personalized Approaches to Improving Gut Health

Let's go back to that intricate dance between what we eat, our gut, and our mental well-being. Imagine a world where your diet isn't a generic blueprint but a personalized guide to gut health and mental bliss. Intriguing, right?

I've had my share of battles with digestive issues—bloating, occasional discomfort, and unpredictable tummy troubles. It got me thinking: What if there's more to gut health than a one-size-fits-all approach?

Our guts are as unique as our fingerprints. What works for one may not work for another. It's like trying to force Cinderella's glass slipper onto everyone, a charming idea, but not practical.

Enter personalized nutrition. It considers your quirks, preferences, and even those guilty pleasures that make life delicious. It's about crafting a menu that suits your gut, promoting a symphony of good bacteria while bidding farewell to the mischief-makers.

Now, onto the link between personalized nutrition and mental health. Stress can send your stomach into somersaults. It's a gut feeling (pun intended). Remember, the gut and the brain are in constant communication, influencing moods and mental well-being. Individualized dietary plans bring much-needed support to mental health management. Crafting a daily menu that nourishes your body and shields you against modern stressors empowers you to face life's challenges.

I have also battled stress and mood swings. Aligning my diet with what my body and mind craved lifted the fog. It wasn't an overnight miracle but a gradual transformation, leaving me feeling grounded and emotionally resilient.

So, the takeaway here is simple: your gut is unique, and so should be your approach to nourishing it. Embrace the power of personalized nutrition, not as a trend but as a key to unlocking a happier gut and a more balanced mind. Your body is whispering its needs; all you have to do is listen, one personalized bite at a time.

Create a Gut-Friendly Diet Plan

Now that we've discussed the benefits of tailoring your nutrition to your needs, let's create a meal plan that's kind to your gut. Think of it as a personalized approach to nourishing both your body and mind.

Understand Your Body

- Reflect on how different foods impact you. Take note of any discomfort, bloating, or sensitivities.

- Consider any known food allergies or sensitivities you may have.

Embrace Whole Foods

- Fill your plate with a variety of vegetables and fruits. They're rich in fiber, which is crucial for gut health.

- Choose whole grains such as quinoa, brown rice, and oats for sustained energy and digestive support.

Include Probiotics

- Integrate probiotic-rich foods like yogurt, kefir, sauerkraut, and kimchi. These contribute beneficial bacteria to your gut.

- Explore different fermented foods to find what suits your taste.

Choose Lean Proteins

- Select lean protein sources like chicken, fish, tofu, and legumes. They're gentler on digestion and provide essential amino acids.

- Consider incorporating plant-based protein options for diversity.

Embrace Healthy Fats
- Incorporate sources of healthy fats like avocados, nuts, seeds, and olive oil. They aid in nutrient absorption and support overall well-being.
- Limit saturated and trans fats commonly found in processed foods.

Prioritize Hydration
- Stay adequately hydrated throughout the day. Hydration supports digestion and facilitates nutrient transport.
- Experiment with herbal teas and infused water for added flavor.

Practice Mindful Eating
- Eat slowly and savor each bite. Thoroughly chewing your food aids digestion.
- Consider keeping a food journal to track how your body responds to various meals.

Minimize Processed Foods and Sugars
- Reduce intake of processed foods, which often contain additives that may not be gut-friendly.
- Be mindful of added sugars; opt for natural sweeteners like honey or maple syrup.

Experiment and Listen to Your Body

- Introduce new foods gradually and observe your body's responses.

- Be open to adjusting your meal plan based on what makes you feel the best.

Seek Professional Advice
- If you have specific dietary concerns or health conditions, consult with a registered dietitian or healthcare professional for more personalized guidance.

Remember, this is your journey to a healthier gut. It's about discovering what works uniquely for you. Enjoy your nourishing meals!

Chapter Five

Lifestyle Choices for Digestive Wellness

Did you know that, on average, 60 to 70 million Americans battle digestive woes? It's time to rewrite your gut's story. For the 73 percent of women facing pre-period digestive blues, and everyone else with a glum tum, this chapter unveils the power of lifestyle choices.

Practical Techniques for Supporting the Gut

While sharing insights on mindful eating is important, it's evident that our bodies require more than that to foster digestive wellness. Let's explore practical techniques that extend beyond our plates, becoming allies in the quest for a healthier gut.

Engage in Purposeful Movement: I've personally found solace in the gentle rhythm of movement. Exercise goes beyond physical sculpting; it's a catalyst for gut health. Simple practices like walking, yoga, or light stretches can stimulate digestion and alleviate bloating.

Harness the Power of Breath: Breathing transcends a reflex. It is also a powerful tool for gut harmony. Mindful breathing techniques, such as diaphragmatic breathing, not only reduce stress but also enhance the parasympathetic nervous system, fostering optimal digestion.

Embrace Stress-Relief Rituals: Stress silently disrupts digestive peace. Through personal exploration, I've uncovered the profound impact of stress-relief practices. From meditation to a warm bath, discover what resonates with you. A calm mind sets the stage for a calm gut.

Practice Abdominal Self-Massage: Visualize a soothing touch that reaches the depths of your gut. Abdominal self-massage, with gentle, circular motions, can alleviate tension, promote blood flow, and awaken the digestive forces within.

Maintain Posture Awareness: Good posture aligns your internal organs, promoting optimal function. Be mindful of how you sit, stand, and move throughout the day. Let your gut benefit from the advantages of proper alignment.

Prioritize Quality Sleep Rituals: Often overlooked, sleep is a cornerstone of well-being. Prioritize a restful night's sleep to allow your body time to repair and rejuvenate. A well-rested gut is better equipped to tackle the challenges of the day.

Embark on this physical journey with me, where each intentional movement becomes a gesture of care for your gut. These practices, combined with mindful dietary choices, form a harmonious symphony that resonates with the rhythm of digestive well-being.

The Connection between Gut Health and Sleep

In my pursuit of a healthier gut, I've uncovered a critical factor that often goes unnoticed: the significance of getting enough quality sleep. As I delved into the intricate connection between sleep and gut health, it became increasingly clear that the relationship is more profound than I initially thought.

Quality sleep isn't just a luxury; it's a necessity for the well-being of our gut. During the hours we're sleep, our bodies engage in essential repair and rejuvenation processes. This nightly restoration extends its benefits to the gut, contributing to healing, reduced inflammation, and enhanced resilience against digestive issues.

The interdependence between gut health and sleep is fascinating. Not only does sleep nurture the gut, but the state of our gut can also influence the quality of our sleep. Our gut microbes, those tiny inhabitants of our digestive tract, play a crucial role in regulating sleep patterns. The delicate balance of these microbes affects the production of neurotransmitters like serotonin and melatonin, key players in promoting restful sleep.

So, how can we ensure we get enough of this sleep-induced elixir for gut healing? Here are some personal insights I've gathered along the way:

Establish a Consistent Sleep Routine: Like our digestive system, our sleep cycle thrives on regularity. Set a consistent bedtime and wake-up time to sync with your body's internal clock.

Create a Relaxing Bedtime Ritual: Wind down before bed with calming activities. Whether it's reading a book, gentle stretches, or a warm bath, these rituals signal to your body that it's time to prepare for rest.

Mind Your Gut-Friendly Diet: Your daytime eating habits can impact your sleep. Opt for gut-friendly foods, such as fiber-rich fruits and vegetables, and consider a balanced evening meal to avoid disrupting your digestive system during the night.

Limit Stimulants before Bed: Caffeine and electronic devices can interfere with both gut health and sleep. Minimize these stimulants in the hours leading up to your bedtime routine.

Prioritizing sufficient sleep that is high in quality has become a cornerstone of my journey toward optimal gut health. In the quiet moments of the night, the magic unfolds, weaving together the threads of gut healing and peaceful slumber.

Exercise and Digestion

Exercise is a dynamic force that influences the gut in multifaceted ways. One notable benefit is the promotion of a diverse and flourishing gut microbiome. Engaging in regular workouts increases the abundance and variety of beneficial microbes, contributing to a more resilient and balanced gut ecosystem.

Exercise also plays a pivotal role in enhancing gut motility—the rhythmic contraction and relaxation of the intestinal muscles that drive food movement. This not only aids digestion but also helps prevent issues like constipation, fostering a smoother and more efficient gut.

The impact of exercise on emotional resilience adds another layer to this narrative. In my own journey of embracing physical activity, I found that it led to a positive shift in my mood and stress levels. Regular exercise has a profound impact on the release of neurotransmitters like endorphins and serotonin, known as the feel-good chemicals. These neurotransmitters not only uplift mood but also contribute to a more balanced and resilient emotional state.

As we recently delved into, in the realm of gut health, the gut-brain axis takes center stage. This bidirectional communication highway connects the gut and the brain, influencing both digestive processes and emotional well-being. Exercise, it turns out, is a powerful conductor on this axis, fostering a harmonious interplay between the gut and the brain.

As I integrated exercise into my routine, it became more than just a physical practice; it became a sanctuary for emotional release and resilience. The meditative rhythm of a run, the empowering feeling of lifting weights, or the grounding nature of yoga all became avenues for promoting gut health and cultivating emotional strength.

So, how can you embark on this journey of integrating exercise into your life for the betterment of gut health and emotional resilience? Here are a few personal insights:

Find Joy in Movement: Discover physical activities that bring you joy. Whether it's dancing, hiking, or practicing martial arts, choose activities that resonate with you.

Consistency Matters: Aim for regularity rather than intensity. Consistent, moderate exercise has been shown to yield long-term benefits for both gut health and emotional well-being.

Listen to Your Body: Pay attention to how your body responds to different forms of exercise. This mindful approach helps tailor your routine to suit your unique needs.

Combine Aerobic and Strength Training: Incorporating a mix of aerobic exercises and strength training will benefit cardiovascular health and muscle strength while contributing to a well-rounded impact on gut health.

Now that we've looked at how to incorporate exercise into your routine, let's look at the different types of exercise that can be incorporated and the benefits they bring to gut health.

Aerobic Exercise (e.g., Brisk Walking, Jogging, Cycling)

Duration: Aim for at least 30 minutes of moderate-intensity aerobic exercise most days of the week.

Benefits: Aerobic activities stimulate the digestive system, promoting regular bowel movements and reducing the risk of constipation.

Yoga

Duration: A 20- to 30-minute yoga session several times a week will help you feel its benefits the most.

Benefits: Yoga poses, especially those focusing on twisting and bending, can massage the abdominal organs, improving digestion and reducing bloating.

Strength Training (e.g., Weightlifting, Resistance Exercises)

Duration: Include strength training exercises two to three times a week, targeting major muscle groups.

Benefits: Building muscle mass can boost metabolism and promote overall bodily function, including digestion.

Walking after Meals

Duration: A 10- to 15-minute walk after meals can be effective.

Benefits: Walking aids in the movement of food through the digestive tract, helping to prevent indigestion and promoting better nutrient absorption.

High-Intensity Interval Training (HIIT)

Duration: Short, intense bursts of exercise (15 to 30 minutes) interspersed with rest.

Benefits: HIIT can improve overall fitness and may enhance metabolism, contributing to better digestion.

It's important to choose activities that you enjoy and can maintain consistently. Always consult with a healthcare professional or fitness expert before starting a new exercise regimen, especially if you have any pre-existing health conditions.

Tailoring your exercise routine to your preferences and physical condition will make it more sustainable, ensuring that movement becomes a positive and regular contributor to your digestive well-being.

Real Life Changes from Exercise

Eva's Journey to Improved Digestion through Running

Eva had been grappling with sluggish digestion and frequent indigestion for years. Tired of the cycle of discomfort, she decided to make running a regular part of her routine. As she started incorporating running into her life, Eva not only experienced improvements in her cardiovascular health but also noticed a significant positive change in her digestive well-being. The rhythmic motion of running seemed to invigorate her digestive system, leading to more regular bowel movements and a visible reduction in bloating.

Jake's Digestive Miracle with HIIT Workouts

Jake, a fitness enthusiast, always enjoyed high-intensity workouts. Little did he know that these intense sessions would bring unexpected relief to his digestive problems. Dealing with occasional constipation and discomfort, Jake found that his commitment to vigorous exercise became a game-changer. The increased blood flow and elevated heart rate seemed to enhance gut motility (the ability of organisms and fluid to move or get around), providing a natural solution to his digestive woes. Jake's experience highlights how intense workouts can positively impact both physical fitness and digestive comfort.

Yoga and Gut Harmony

Before we move on from exercise, it's important to spend a little more time focusing on yoga. Gut harmony and yoga are closely linked, in that they both play vital roles in overall well-being. See the following for various ways the gut and the mind are connected:

Stress Reduction

Yoga is recognized for its stress-reducing benefits, which is important for the gut because stress is known to impact the gut negatively through issues like inflammation and changes in gut microbiota. Practices such as deep breathing and meditation in yoga activate the relaxation response, reducing stress levels and contributing to a healthier gut environment.

Mind-Body Connection

The gut-brain axis is influenced by emotional and psychological factors. Yoga emphasizes the mind-body connection, encouraging practitioners to be present and mindful during their practice.

Physical Movement

Yoga involves physical postures and movements that stimulate the digestive organs. Twisting poses, for instance, can massage the digestive tract and improve digestion. This helps regulate bowel movements and prevent constipation, promoting a healthier gut.

Breath Control (Pranayama)

The breath control exercises practiced in yoga directly impact the autonomic nervous system, which influences the balance between the sympathetic and parasympathetic branches. Deep diaphragmatic breathing in yoga activates the parasympathetic nervous system, enhancing digestion and nutrient absorption by promoting a state of relaxation.

Holistic Wellness

Holistic wellness is crucial for maintaining a healthy gut. Yoga promotes this by addressing mental, emotional, and physical well-being.

While yoga can contribute to gut harmony, individual responses may vary. Adopting a comprehensive approach to health, including a balanced diet, regular exercise, and proper hydration alongside yoga practices, can maximize benefits for gut health. Always consult healthcare professionals for personalized advice, especially if you have specific gut-related concerns or conditions (Jain, 2023).

Stories of Gut-Health Victories from Yoga

Eleana's Stress Relief

Eleana, a twenty-eight-year-old professional juggling a demanding job, struggled with persistent digestive issues. Seeking relief, she turned to yoga. Consistent practice, focusing on stress-reducing poses and mindful breathing, brought a notable improvement in her digestion. The mind-body connection fostered by yoga became a key element in Eleana's overall well-being.

Tom's IBS Management

Tom, a thirty-eight-year-old with irritable bowel syndrome (IBS), found solace in yoga. Initially hesitant, he began with beginner-friendly classes emphasizing controlled breathing and gentle movements. As he maintained a regular practice, Tom experienced reduced stress levels and a significant decrease in the frequency and severity of his digestive issues. Yoga became a vital part of his daily routine, providing both serenity and digestive comfort.

Yoga Poses That Aid Digestion and Reduce Stress

I've discovered a set of yoga poses that have been beneficial for improving digestion and alleviating specific digestive issues. Here's a brief guide to some of my favorite poses:

1. *Seated Side Bend (Parsva Sukhasana):* A beginner-friendly move that stretches obliques, belly muscles, and the upper and lower back, providing relief from bloating and gas.

2. *Seated Twist (Ardha Matsyendrasana):* This twisting pose promotes bowel regularity, aiding the small and large intestines. It's effective in reducing bloating and enhancing digestion.

3. *Supine Spinal Twist (Supta Matsyendrasana):* Ideal for stretching the lower back and increasing spinal mobility, believed to alleviate constipation, bloating, and support general digestion.

4. *Knees to Chest (Apanasana):* A gentle movement that relaxes and relieves lower back strain, with claims of massaging the

large intestine to promote bowel movements.

5. *Cat-Cow (Marjaryasana-Bitilasana):* Transitioning between cat pose and cow pose, these stretches improve circulation and gently massage organs to promote gut peristalsis.

6. *Cobra Pose (Bhujangasana):* This pose mimics a cobra's upright position, stretches belly muscles, improves posture, and is believed to support overall digestion (Sullivan, 2021).

Incorporating these poses into my routine has been a game-changer for my digestive well-being. Remember to practice each pose mindfully, focusing on deep breaths and maintaining proper form.

Smoking and Your Gut

Smoking has detrimental effects on the digestive system, increasing the chances of heartburn, peptic ulcers, and complications in their treatment. It also raises the risk of Crohn's disease, gallstones, and exacerbates liver disease and pancreatitis. Furthermore, there is a correlation between smoking and cancers in digestive organs, including the head, neck, stomach, pancreas, and colon.

All in all, quitting smoking is crucial to reducing the risk of various digestive disorders, cancers, and associated health complications. Seeking professional assistance can be beneficial in the journey of quitting to improve overall digestive health.

Alcohol Consumption

Excessive alcohol consumption can have a range of negative impacts on gut health, extending beyond common issues, such as hangovers. While moderate drinking (up to one drink a day for women and two drinks a day for men) is generally considered safe, surpassing these limits can lead to potential problems. These include:

Acid Reflux: Alcohol relaxes the lower esophageal sphincter, causing acid reflux or heartburn. Persistent acid reflux may lead to more severe conditions like Barrett's esophagus or esophageal cancer.

Diarrhea: Alcohol disrupts the balance of gut bacteria, promoting inflammation and leading to a leaky gut. This condition allows toxins to enter the bloodstream, contributing to diarrhea.

Gastritis: Excessive alcohol disrupts mucus production in the stomach, causing inflammation known as gastritis. Repeated episodes can lead to ulcers, anemia, or stomach cancer.

Bloating: Alcohol affects sugar digestion and alters the balance of gut bacteria, leading to bloating. Beer is more commonly associated with this issue compared to wine or spirits.

Liver Damage: Heavy alcohol use can result in alcoholic fatty liver disease, leading to liver failure, cancer, or cirrhosis over time. Early detection through routine bloodwork allows for reversibility with lifestyle changes.

Pancreatic Damage: Alcohol can damage the pancreas, causing inflammation (pancreatitis). This condition can be life-threatening, especially for heavy drinkers and smokers, increasing the risk of organ failure and long-term complications, such as diabetes and pancreatic cancer.

Treatment for alcohol-induced pancreatitis can be administered in various ways, including IV fluids, electrolyte replacement, tube feeding, and counseling for alcohol cessation. Severe cases may necessitate surgery and involve a lengthy recovery, with potential long-term complications. It is crucial to be aware of these risks and seek medical advice for moderation or cessation of alcohol consumption.

The Impact of Antibiotics on Gut Flora

Antibiotics play a crucial role in treating bacterial infections but can disrupt the delicate balance of gut flora. These medications, designed to target specific bacteria, often affect both harmful and beneficial microbes in the gastrointestinal tract, leading to a potential reduction in microbial diversity. This disturbance may result in various digestive issues and an increased vulnerability to infections.

Prolonged antibiotic use could also have lasting effects on gut flora, potentially contributing to conditions like irritable bowel syndrome (IBS) or inflammatory bowel disease (IBD).

To mitigate these effects, it is important to use antibiotics judiciously and consider counter-measures, such as incorporating probiotics or prebiotics post-treatment, to support the restoration of a healthy gut microbiome.

Food Intolerances and Sensitivities

Recognizing and addressing food intolerances can pose challenges, yet it is crucial for enhancing one's health. Distinguishing itself from allergies, food intolerance doesn't involve the immune system but arises from difficulties in digesting specific foods, like lactose.

Causes include insufficient digestive enzymes, potential nutritional deficiencies, prolonged illnesses, or sensitivities to certain foods like gluten. Precise diagnosis requires assessment by specialists, such as allergists or dietitians, and typically involves blood and skin tests. Once identified, managing food intolerances involves steering clear of problematic foods, using digestive enzyme supplements, and monitoring nutritional intake.

Adopting lifestyle changes, including stress reduction, regular exercise, and mindful eating, can alleviate symptoms and promote overall well-being. Taking a proactive stance and seeking professional guidance when necessary are pivotal steps in navigating food intolerances.

Common Symptoms of Food Intolerances

Food intolerances can lead to various uncomfortable symptoms, such as bloating, gas, and abdominal pain. These symptoms may resemble those of conditions like inflammatory bowel disease and celiac disease.

The manifestations of food intolerance can differ among individuals and may be influenced by factors like the quantity and type of food consumed. Digestive issues are common, but skin and joint symptoms can also arise. Symptoms typically emerge within 30 minutes to 48 hours after consuming the problematic food.

Common intolerances, such as lactose intolerance, affect a significant portion of the global population. Naturally occurring chemicals in food, such as glutamate, salicylates, and amines, contribute to intolerance.

Beyond gastrointestinal symptoms, other effects may include nausea, vomiting, acid reflux, migraines, fatigue, and irritability, which highlights the diverse impact of food intolerance on overall well-being.

Elimination Diets for Identifying Food Intolerances and Sensitivities

An elimination diet can be effective in addressing inflammation and gastrointestinal issues by temporarily removing specific foods. There are various approaches to this diet, such as Whole30, autoimmune protocol, low-FODMAP, and Specific Carbohydrate Diet, among others, each with its own set of guidelines. Some diets also recommend reducing sugar, caffeine, and alcohol intake.

During the elimination phase, which typically lasts one to three months, strict adherence is crucial to accurately assess improvements in symptoms. It's important to note that inflammatory reactions to certain foods may persist for up to two weeks after ingestion. Therefore, maintaining strict compliance during this phase is essential for optimal results.

Equally important is the reintroduction phase, where each eliminated food is systematically reintroduced, following a protocol of incremental intake over two to three days. This is proceeded by an observation phase for three to four days. Keeping a food and symptom diary helps track unexpected benefits or adverse reactions.

Symptoms to monitor during reintroduction include skin changes, mood swings, headaches, sleep disturbances, nasal congestion, fluid retention, joint or muscle pain, fatigue, and gastrointestinal issues. The goal is to gather comprehensive knowledge about how different foods impact individual well-being, enabling informed decisions on whether to avoid certain foods or consume them in moderation.

After completing the elimination diet, it is advisable to adhere to good nutrition principles by incorporating a variety of whole-plant foods, while at the same time limiting added-sugar and processed foods. This ensures a balanced and healthy dietary approach moving forward.

How to Manage Food Intolerances in Daily Life

Identify Triggers: Work with a professional to pinpoint trigger foods through tests or an elimination diet.

Educate Yourself: Learn about alternative ingredients and read labels to avoid hidden intolerant-inducing components.

Meal Planning: Plan meals, opting for homemade options to control ingredients.

Communication: Communicate intolerance to others, especially when dining out.

Choose Whole Foods: Prioritize unprocessed options, such as fresh fruits, vegetables, lean proteins, and whole grains.

Experiment with Cooking: Try different cooking methods, and use herbs and spices for flavor without triggering intolerances.

Read Labels: Thoroughly read food labels to identify potential allergens or intolerant-inducing ingredients.

Carry Safe Snacks: Keep safe snacks on hand for situations with limited food options.

Stay Informed: Stay updated on new products and changes in ingredient formulations.

Consult Professionals: Regularly consult with healthcare professionals or dietitians to ensure nutritional needs are met.

Gut Reset

A gut reset involves making intentional dietary and lifestyle changes to promote a healthier gut microbiome. This typically includes eliminating potential irritants, introducing gut-friendly foods, incorporating probiotics, staying hydrated, and managing stress. The duration varies, and consulting healthcare professionals for personalized guidance is advisable. The goal is to support digestion, address gut-related issues, and enhance overall well-being.

Success Stories

Paul's Achievements

Paul successfully lowered his blood pressure, increased focus, and achieved weight loss through a gut reset. Despite facing a demanding job and a hectic lifestyle, the reset reduced his blood pressure and left him feeling more energized and significantly sharper. Additionally, he experienced significant weight loss.

Megan's Progress

Megan found relief beyond prescribed medications for her chronic stomach conditions through a gut reset. Dealing with Barrett's, esophagitis, and reflux disease, along with insomnia, aches, and low energy, Megan decided to try the cleanse based on a friend's suggestion. To her surprise, the reset alleviated her stomach issues more effectively than the prescribed medication and improved her sleep and overall well-being.

The Benefits and Limitations of a Gut Reset
Benefits of a Gut Reset:

Improved Digestive Health: A gut reset can help alleviate digestive issues, such as bloating, gas, and irregular bowel movements. It allows the digestive system to recalibrate and function more efficiently.

Balanced Gut Microbiome: Resetting the gut often involves introducing probiotics and prebiotics, fostering a balanced and diverse gut microbiome. This can positively impact overall health, including immune function and mental well-being.

Increased Nutrient Absorption: A healthier gut environment enhances the absorption of nutrients from food, ensuring that the body receives the necessary vitamins and minerals for optimal functioning.

Weight Management: Some individuals experience weight loss as a result of a gut reset. This may be attributed to improved digestion, reduced inflammation, and better metabolism.

Enhanced Energy Levels: By promoting efficient digestion and nutrient absorption, a gut reset can lead to increased energy levels. Individuals often report feeling more vibrant and alert.

Improved Mental Health: Because of the link between the gut and mental health, a gut reset may contribute to improved mood and cognitive function, although individual responses vary.

Limitations of a Gut Reset:

Individual Variability: Responses to a gut reset can vary significantly among individuals. What works well for one person may not yield the same results for another, as each person's microbiome and health conditions are unique.

Temporary Effects: The benefits of a gut reset may be temporary if underlying lifestyle factors, such as poor dietary choices or high stress levels, are not addressed in the long term. Maintenance of a healthy gut requires ongoing lifestyle choices.

Potential Discomfort: Some individuals may experience discomfort or mild side effects during the initial phases of a gut reset. This can include changes in bowel habits, bloating, or gas. These symptoms are often transient but are worth mentioning.

Consultation Requirement: Before undertaking a gut reset, individuals with pre-existing health conditions should consult with healthcare professionals. This is crucial to ensure that the reset aligns with their specific health needs and doesn't pose any risks.

A gut reset can offer various benefits, particularly in improving digestive health and promoting overall well-being. However, it is essential to approach it with an understanding of individual variability and the need for sustained healthy habits.

Step-by-Step Guide to a Safe Gut Reset

1. *Consult a Professional:*

- Seek advice from a healthcare professional before making any significant changes.

2. *Gradual Diet Changes:*
- Increase fiber intake with fruits, vegetables, and whole grains.

- Include probiotic-rich foods or supplements.

- Stay hydrated with plenty of water.

3. *Elimination Phase:*
- Reduce processed and sugary foods.

- Consider an elimination diet under professional guidance.

4. *Mindful Eating:*
- Chew thoroughly.

- Establish regular mealtimes.

- Eat without distractions.

5. *Stress Management:*
- Engage in regular exercise.

- Practice mindfulness activities like meditation or yoga.

6. *Sleep Health:*
- Maintain a consistent sleep schedule.

- Establish a relaxing bedtime routine.

7. *Reintroduction:*
    - Gradually reintroduce eliminated foods one at a time.
    - Monitor your body's response.

8. *Long-Term Maintenance:*
    - Adopt a balanced, varied diet for sustained gut health.
    - Regularly assess and adjust your lifestyle.

9. *Regular Check-ins:*
    - Schedule follow-ups with a healthcare professional.
    - Discuss progress and make adjustments as needed (Skwiat, 2019).

Remember, personalization and professional guidance are essential for a safe and effective gut reset.

The Role of Healthcare Professionals in Guiding a Gut Reset

Take care when choosing a healthcare professional because they play a pivotal role in guiding a safe and effective gut reset. Through individualized assessments, they will tailor the reset plan to your unique health profile, identifying underlying issues and any potential risks. Then, armed with evidence-based practices, they will offer recommendations for gradual dietary changes, help you monitor your progress, and make any necessary adjustments.

Collaboration with a specialist will ensure you receive comprehensive care that prioritizes the individual's well-being. The specialist will also educate and empower you, fostering sustainable habits for long-term gut health beyond the reset period.

Gut Reset Plan

Here's a straightforward plan for resetting your gut that integrates fundamental principles to support digestive health. Keep in mind that individual reactions can differ, so consulting with a healthcare professional before making significant dietary changes is recommended.

Hydration:

- Begin your day with a glass of water to initiate hydration.

- Strive to consume at least eight glasses of water throughout the day.

Fiber-Rich Foods:

- Include an assortment of fruits, vegetables, whole grains, and legumes in your meals.

- Fiber promotes digestive regularity and nurtures beneficial gut bacteria.

Probiotic Foods:

- Integrate probiotic-rich foods like yogurt, kefir, sauerkraut, or kimchi into your diet.

- If necessary, consider a high-quality probiotic supplement.

Limit Processed Foods:

- Reduce the intake of processed and sugary foods.

- Opt for whole, unprocessed foods to foster a diverse microbiome.

Mindful Eating:

- Engage in mindful eating by thoroughly chewing food and relishing each bite.

- Steer clear of distractions, such as screens, during meals.

Herbal Teas:
- Include soothing herbal teas, like peppermint or ginger, known for aiding digestion.

Limit Caffeine and Alcohol:
- Diminish the consumption of caffeinated beverages and alcohol, recognizing their potential impact on gut health.

Regular Meals and Snacks:
- Set consistent mealtimes to uphold a regular eating schedule.
- Incorporate healthy snacks, if necessary, to prevent extended periods without food.

Physical Activity:
- Involve yourself in regular physical activity to support overall well-being, including digestive health.

Adequate Sleep:
- Ensure you get sufficient, quality sleep by adhering to a regular sleep schedule and engaging in healthy sleep practices.

Stress Management:
- Include stress-reducing activities, like meditation, deep breathing, or yoga, in your routine.

Reintroduction and Observation:
- After a few weeks, gradually reintroduce eliminated foods and observe how your body reacts.

Always pay attention to your body's signals and make adjustments based on your individual needs and preferences. If you have any underlying health conditions or concerns, seeking personalized guidance from a healthcare professional is recommended.

Revitalize 360

Boost Immunity, Ignite Wellbeing, & Transform Your Gut Health for a Harmonious, Radiant You!

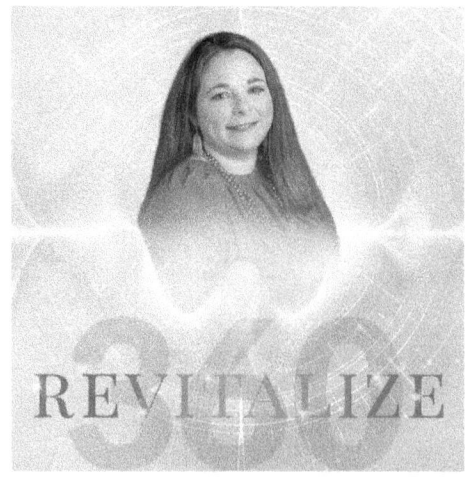

Dr. Ashley's 90-day Gut Reset Program

If you're ready to supercharge your gut health with personalized guidance, my Group Gut Healing Program is designed for you. Join a community of like-minded individuals on a transformative journey to optimal gut wellness.

- Decrease symptoms of bloating, gas, constipation, diarrhea
- Improve nutrient absorption to support body function
- Reduce fatigue and improve energy levels to increase activity and engagement
- Establish more mental clarity
- Boost immune function
- Improve skin blemishes
- Reduce chronic inflammation

Program Includes:
- Lab diagnostics
- 1:1 lab review
- 30-day detox
- 90-day replenishment
- Complete PDF guide

- Unlimited group access: No expiration, Continued support, Q & A calls, Topic discussions

Check it out HERE!

https://ashleysullivanonline.com/products-and-services/revitalize-360-product-page/

Chapter Six

Healing Herbs and Remedies

> *"All those spices and herbs in your spice rack can do more than provide calorie-free, natural flavorings to enhance and make food delicious. They're also an incredible source of antioxidants and help rev up your metabolism and improve your health at the same time."* - Suzanne Somers

Chapter 6 is all about simple and natural ways to keep your stomach healthy with herbs and remedies that come from nature to support your gut. The goal is to help you learn about these natural options, so that you feel confident using them to improve your own gut health.

Herbal Allies for the Gut

Numerous herbs are recognized for their potential advantages in promoting a healthy digestive system. These herbs are believed to contribute to the alleviation of digestive problems, reduction of inflammation, and the support of a thriving gut microbiome. The following herbs are commonly associated with promoting gut health:

Peppermint (Mentha piperita)

Benefits: Eases symptoms of irritable bowel syndrome (IBS), including abdominal pain and bloating. It possesses anti-inflammatory and antispasmodic properties.

Ginger (Zingiber officinale)

Benefits: Facilitates digestion, alleviates nausea, and may assist with indigestion. Ginger is known for its anti-inflammatory and antioxidant properties.

Turmeric (Curcuma longa)

Benefits: Contains curcumin, which exhibits anti-inflammatory and antioxidant properties. It may aid in reducing symptoms associated with inflammatory bowel diseases (IBD).

Chamomile (Matricaria chamomilla)

Benefits: Soothes the digestive tract, diminishes indigestion, and may alleviate symptoms of IBS. Chamomile has anti-inflammatory and calming effects.

Fennel (Foeniculum vulgare)

Benefits: Alleviates bloating, gas, and indigestion. Fennel seeds have historical use as a digestive aid.

Licorice (Glycyrrhiza glabra)

Benefits: Assists in soothing the stomach lining and may be utilized to address symptoms of heartburn and ulcers. It exhibits anti-inflammatory properties.

Aloe Vera (Aloe barbadensis miller)

Benefits: Aloe vera gel may aid in managing digestive issues like constipation and irritable bowel syndrome. It possesses anti-inflammatory and soothing properties.

Dandelion (Taraxacum officinale)

Benefits: Supports liver health, indirectly benefiting digestion. Dandelion root is occasionally used as a mild laxative and digestive aid.

Slippery Elm (Ulmus rubra)

Benefits: Soothes the digestive tract and may be helpful for conditions such as gastritis and acid reflux. It forms a protective layer in the digestive tract.

Marshmallow Root (Althaea officinalis)

Benefits: Contains mucilage, offering soothing and protective effects on the digestive tract. It may be employed for conditions like gastritis and heartburn.

Lemon Balm (Melissa officinalis)

Benefits: Exhibits mild calming effects and may assist with indigestion and gas. Lemon balm promotes relaxation, which is advantageous for digestion.

Cinnamon (Cinnamomum verum)

Benefits: May contribute to regulating blood sugar levels and improving insulin sensitivity, indirectly benefiting gut health.

Coriander (Coriandrum sativum)

Benefits: Aids digestion, reduces gas, and may alleviate symptoms of irritable bowel syndrome (IBS). Coriander has anti-inflammatory properties.

Mint (Mentha spp.)

Benefits: Eases indigestion, reduces gas, and may provide relief from symptoms of IBS. Mint also has a calming effect on the digestive tract.

Rosemary (Rosmarinus officinalis)

Benefits: Supports digestion, reduces bloating, and has antimicrobial properties that may contribute to a healthy gut environment.

Oregano (Origanum vulgare)

Benefits: Possesses antimicrobial and anti-inflammatory properties, which can support a balanced gut microbiome and alleviate digestive discomfort.

Holy Basil (Ocimum sanctum)

Benefits: Known for its adaptogenic properties, holy basil may help the body manage stress, which can have a positive impact on digestive health.

Thyme (Thymus vulgaris)

Benefits: Supports digestion, reduces inflammation, and has antimicrobial properties that may aid in maintaining a healthy balance of gut bacteria.

Rose Hip (Rosa canina)

Benefits: Rich in antioxidants, rose hip may contribute to reducing inflammation in the digestive system and support overall gut health.

Nettle (Urtica dioica)

Benefits: Supports the liver and may indirectly benefit digestion. Nettle tea is often used as a gentle digestive tonic.

Cumin (Cuminum cyminum)

Benefits: Aids digestion, reduces bloating, and may help alleviate symptoms of indigestion. Cumin also has antimicrobial properties.

Astragalus (Astragalus membranaceus)

Benefits: Known for its immune-boosting properties, astragalus may contribute to overall gut health by supporting the body's defenses.

Catnip (Nepeta cataria)

Benefits: Has calming effects on the digestive system, reducing indigestion and bloating. Catnip tea is commonly used for digestive comfort (*Explore The 12 Best Herbs for Digestion*, 2022).

Vitamins

Vitamins, minerals, and antioxidants play critical roles in supporting optimal gut function. Listed within this section are key nutrients that are particularly important for promoting gut health. Recommended dosages and usage guidelines are also included.

1. Vitamin D:

- Role: Essential for regulating the immune system, so it has the potential to reduce gut inflammation.

- Additional Benefits: Facilitates calcium absorption, contributing to the maintenance of a healthy gut lining.

- Recommended Daily Allowance (RDA): It is advisable to adhere to the daily intake levels recommended by health authorities to support overall health.

- 2. Vitamin C:

- Role: Functions as an antioxidant, playing a pivotal role in supporting the immune system.

- Additional Benefits: May help mitigate oxidative stress within the gut.

- RDA: Meeting the recommended daily intake of vitamin C is crucial for its various health-promoting effects.

- 3. Vitamin A:

- Role: Critical for preserving the integrity of the gut lining.

- Additional Benefits: Supports the health of mucous membranes within the digestive system.

- RDA: Adhering to the recommended daily intake of Vitamin A is important for sustaining gut health and overall well-being.

- 4. Vitamin E:

- Role: Functions as an antioxidant, providing protection against oxidative damage to the gut lining.

- RDA: Ensuring an adequate intake of Vitamin E is essential in harnessing its protective effects on the digestive system.

Understanding the significance of these nutrients in the context of digestive health underscores the importance of maintaining a balanced and varied diet. Including a diverse range of foods rich in these vitamins contributes to the upkeep of a healthy gut and overall well-being.

Minerals

1. Calcium:

- Role: Essential for muscle function within the digestive tract.

- Additional Benefits: Maintains the tight junctions of the gut lining, contributing to the overall structural integrity of the digestive system.

1. Magnesium:

- Role: Supports muscle contractions in the digestive system.

- Additional Benefits: Regulates bowel movements, aiding in the overall coordination and efficiency of the digestive process.

1. Zinc:

- Role: Contributes to maintaining the integrity of the gut lining.

- Additional Benefits: Supports immune function, playing a vital role in the body's defense mechanisms related to digestive health.

1. Iron:

- Role: Essential for the formation of hemoglobin, which transports oxygen to cells, including those in the digestive tract.

- Additional Benefits: Supports overall energy metabolism, crucial for the efficient functioning of digestive organs.

1. Potassium:

- Role: Facilitates proper muscle contractions, including those involved in digestion.

- Additional Benefits: Maintains fluid balance, aiding in the prevention of dehydration, which is important for healthy digestion.

1. Selenium:

- Role: Functions as an antioxidant, protecting cells in the digestive system from oxidative damage.

- Additional Benefits: Supports the immune system and may contribute to the prevention of inflammation in the digestive tract.

1. Copper:

- Role: Plays a role in the formation of connective tissue, which is essential for the structural integrity of the digestive organs.

- Additional Benefits: Contributes to the absorption and utilization of iron, supporting overall digestive function.

1. Manganese:

- Role: Participates in the metabolism of amino acids and carbohydrates, supporting the energy needs of digestive tissues.

- Additional Benefits: Acts as an antioxidant, helping to protect cells in the digestive system from oxidative stress.

Incorporating a diverse range of nutrient-rich foods into your diet ensures an adequate intake of these minerals, promoting digestive health and overall well-being.

Antioxidants

Antioxidants play a crucial role in promoting digestive health by counteracting oxidative stress and inflammation. Here are several antioxidants, each with unique contributions to safeguarding the gut:

1. **Glutathione:**

- A potent antioxidant known for its ability to protect the gut lining from oxidative stress and inflammation.

- Glutathione serves as a key defender against harmful free radicals, thereby supporting the overall well-being of the digestive system.

1. **Quercetin:**

- Found in foods like apples, onions, and berries, quercetin is an antioxidant with potential anti-inflammatory properties.

- Its presence in various fruits and vegetables highlights its role in mitigating inflammation within the gut, contributing to digestive wellness.

1. **Polyphenols:**

- These antioxidants, abundant in foods like green tea, red wine, and dark chocolate, play a role in supporting a diverse and healthy gut microbiome.

- Polyphenols contribute to the overall balance of gut bacteria, fostering a microbiome that is conducive to optimal digestive function.

1. **Beta-carotene:**

- An antioxidant that can be converted into vitamin A, playing a vital role in maintaining the health of the gut lining.

- Beta-carotene's conversion into vitamin A underscores its significance in preserving the integrity of the gut lining, essential for overall digestive well-being.

1. **Vitamin C (Ascorbic Acid):**

- An antioxidant found in citrus fruits, strawberries, and bell peppers, vitamin C supports immune function and helps combat oxidative stress in the digestive system.

- Beyond its well-known immune-boosting properties, vitamin C contributes to a healthy gut environment by neutralizing free radicals.

1. **Resveratrol:**

- An antioxidant present in red grapes and berries, resveratrol may have anti-inflammatory effects and, therefore, contribute to gut health.

- Resveratrol's inclusion in the diet, often associated with moderate red wine consumption, provides an additional layer of antioxidant protection for the digestive system.

Incorporating a variety of antioxidant-rich foods into your diet ensures a comprehensive approach to supporting digestive health, as these antioxidants collectively contribute to the body's defense against oxidative challenges.

The Role of Fiber in Gut Health

Fiber is essential for maintaining gut health and overall well-being, impacting digestive processes and the balance of gut microbiota. There are two types:

1. **Insoluble fiber:** Found in whole grains, nuts, seeds, and fruit / vegetable skins, prevents constipation by adding bulk to stool; and

2. **Soluble fiber:** Present in oats, legumes, fruits, and vegetables. It undergoes fermentation, producing short-chain fatty acids (SCFAs) with health benefits. SCFAs support the gut barrier, foster beneficial bacteria growth, manage blood sug-

ar levels, and contribute to weight management by inducing satiety.

Certain fiber-rich foods also possess anti-inflammatory properties, potentially reducing gut and body inflammation and lowering the risk of colorectal cancer. To optimize gut health, gradually incorporate a variety of fiber-rich foods, and consider seeking personalized dietary advice from healthcare professionals or registered dietitians (*Dietary Fiber: Essential for a Healthy Diet*, n.d.).

As discussed in previous chapters, prebiotics and probiotics are also crucial for gut health. Probiotics are live beneficial bacteria that enhance gut health by maintaining a balanced microbiota, while prebiotics are non-digestible fibers that nourish these beneficial bacteria, promoting their growth. Together, they contribute to a healthy gut environment.

Even though your gut is an internal organ, and we are still learning a lot about what goes on inside it, the condition of your gut health can significantly impact how you look on the outside. So, the next chapter will focus on the impact of your gut health on your skin as well as your immunity.

Help Transform Lives

Review Understanding Leaky Gut & Hormonal Health!

Unlock the Power of Generosity

"Money can't buy happiness, but sharing knowledge can." - Dr. Ashley Sullivan

People who share knowledge without expecting anything in return tend to lead happier, healthier lives. So, let's aim for that during our time together.

You can make a real difference. To do that, I have a simple question for you ...

Would you be willing to assist someone you haven't met, even if you never received recognition for it? Who is this person, you wonder? They are much like you, or at least like you used to be—seeking information, wanting to make a positive change, and needing guidance.

Our mission is to make the essential information about leaky gut and digestive health accessible to everyone. Everything I do revolves around that mission. And the only way for me to achieve that is by reaching ... well ... everyone.

This is where your help comes in. Most people do, indeed, judge a book by its cover (and its reviews). So, here's my request on behalf of a struggling individual in search of knowledge about digestive health: Please assist that curious learner by leaving a review for this book.

Your gift costs no money and takes less than 60 seconds, but it can change a fellow seeker's life forever. Your review could help ...

- one more person to make informed health decisions.

- one more family adopt healthier habits.

- one more individual regain control of their well-being; or

- one more friend to share valuable insights.

To experience the joy of making a positive impact and genuinely helping someone, all you need to do—in less than 60 seconds—is leave a review.

Simply scan the QR code below to leave your review:

I'm excited to continue guiding you toward understanding leaky gut and digestive health in faster and easier ways than you can imagine. You'll appreciate the practical insights and strategies I'm about to share in the upcoming chapters.

Thank you sincerely. Now, let's return to our journey of discovery.

Your biggest supporter, **Dr. Ashley.**

P.S. Fun Fact: If you share valuable information, you become more valuable to others. If you believe this book will help another seeker, pass it along—it might just be the knowledge they're looking for.

Chapter Seven

The Impact of Gut Health on Skin and Immunity

"*A healthy outside starts from the inside.*" - Robert Urich

This chapter focuses on the connection between your gut and skin, explaining how what's happening inside your body can affect how your skin looks and feels. By the end of this chapter, you'll have a better understanding of how keeping your gut healthy can lead to better skin and a stronger immune system.

Understanding the Link between Gut Health and Skin

The relationship between gut health and skin is an intriguing and increasingly acknowledged aspect of overall health. The gut, responsible for digestion and maintaining a balance of bacteria, has a significant impact on various aspects of well-being, including skin condition.

Here are some key points that explain the connection between gut health and skin:

- *Microbiome Influence:* The gut hosts trillions of microorganisms, collectively known as the microbiome, which profoundly affect overall health. A balanced microbiome is linked to healthier skin.

- *Inflammation:* Imbalances in the gut microbiome can lead to inflammation, closely tied to skin conditions like acne and eczema. Chronic gut inflammation may contribute to the development or worsening of skin issues.

- *Nutrient Absorption:* The gut absorbs essential nutrients from food, crucial for skin health. Proper gut function ensures the skin receives the necessary nutrients for repair and maintenance.

- *Immune System Support:* Both the gut and skin are vital components of the immune system. A healthy gut supports a robust immune response, helping the body defend against infections and maintain skin integrity.

- *Holistic Approach:* Holistic skincare approaches recognize the significance of addressing internal factors, like diet and gut health, alongside external factors. Focusing on the gut-skin connection allows for a more comprehensive approach to achieving and maintaining healthy skin.

Maintaining a healthy gut not only aids in digestion but also significantly influences skin health. A balanced and thriving gut microbiome contributes to clearer, healthier skin, while imbalances may result in various skin issues. As our understanding of the gut-skin connection expands, so does the importance of holistic approaches to skincare and overall well-being.

The Gut-Skin Axis and Its Impact on Skin Health

The gut-skin axis represents the intricate connection between the gastrointestinal tract and skin health. This bidirectional communication system involves the gut microbiota, immune system, and various signaling molecules, influencing overall well-being, particularly the condition of the skin.

The gut microbiota, consisting of trillions of microorganisms, plays a crucial role in digestion, nutrient absorption, and immune function. Imbalances in the gut microbiota, referred to as dysbiosis, have been associated with skin conditions such as acne, eczema, and psoriasis.

The gut is a key component of the immune system, and disruptions in the microbiota balance can lead to systemic inflammation, a factor linked to various skin disorders. Nutrient absorption in the gut is essential for maintaining skin health, as nutrients contribute to skin structure, repair, and protection.

The gut-skin axis involves complex interactions, including signaling molecules, stress-related hormones, and inflammatory responses that collectively influence skin well-being. Supporting a healthy gut-skin axis through a balanced diet, hydration, stress management, and avoiding trigger foods can contribute to optimal skin health.

Ongoing research aims to deepen our understanding of these complex connections and their implications for dermatological well-being.

The Role of Inflammation in Gut-Skin Interactions

Inflammation plays a vital role in interactions between the gut and the skin, underscoring the intricate connection between the gastrointestinal tract and skin health. This is because the immune system is a central player in this relationship. Disruptions in the gut can lead to systemic inflammation, which influences various aspects of skin health.

Leaky Gut and Systemic Inflammation:
- Disturbances in gut barrier function, commonly referred to as leaky gut, may arise due to imbalances in the gut microbiota, among other factors. This condition allows the entry of toxins, bacteria, and undigested food particles into the bloodstream.

- The presence of these foreign substances in the bloodstream can trigger an immune response, leading to systemic inflammation. This inflammation may impact the skin, potentially contributing to or exacerbating various skin conditions.

Immune System Activation:
- The gut is a significant part of the immune system, as immune cells in the gut interact with the gut microbiota. Imbalances in the microbiota can activate immune responses, resulting in the release of pro-inflammatory cytokines.

- These cytokines, once in circulation, can influence immune responses throughout the body, potentially affecting the skin and contributing to skin inflammation and conditions, like acne, eczema, or psoriasis.

Skin Conditions Linked to Inflammation:
- Chronic inflammation is a common factor in many skin disorders. Conditions such as acne, rosacea, and psoriasis are characterized by inflammation in the skin.

- In the context of the gut-skin axis, inflammation originating in the gut can contribute to the development or exacerbation of these skin conditions. For example, the release of inflammatory mediators can influence the skin's immune responses and lead to the appearance of skin lesions.

Hormonal Influence:
- The gut-skin axis is interconnected with hormonal regulation. Stress-related hormones, such as cortisol, can be released in response to inflammation or gut disturbances.

- Elevated cortisol levels can contribute to skin issues, potentially increasing sebum production and worsening conditions like acne.

Managing Inflammation for Skin Health:
- Addressing inflammation in the gut is a potential strategy for managing skin conditions. This can involve adopting an anti-inflammatory diet, promoting a healthy gut microbiota through probiotics, and managing stress levels.

- Anti-inflammatory agents and lifestyle changes that promote gut health may contribute to reducing inflammation in the skin and improving overall skin health.

Understanding and addressing the role of inflammation in gut-skin interactions can provide valuable insights for developing strategies to manage and prevent skin conditions, emphasizing the importance of a holistic approach to health that considers both gut and skin well-being (*Gut Bacteria Linked to Inflammatory Skin Disease*, 2021).

Gut-Skin Axis and Its Relationship to Eczema

Eczema, also known as atopic dermatitis, is a chronic inflammatory skin condition characterized by red, itchy, and inflamed skin. While the exact cause of eczema is multifactorial and not fully understood, there is increasing evidence to suggest that the gut-skin axis plays a role in its development and exacerbation.

Several mechanisms contribute to the gut-skin axis and its relationship to eczema:

Immune System Crosstalk: An imbalance in immune responses in the gut can affect the skin and vice versa. Dysregulation in immune function may lead to the development of inflammatory skin conditions like eczema.

Gut Microbiota Influence: The microbial community that makes up the gut microbiota play a crucial role in maintaining immune homeostasis. Changes in the gut microbiota composition, often referred to as dysbiosis, have been associated with inflammatory skin conditions, including eczema.

Intestinal Permeability (Leaky Gut): Increased intestinal permeability can allow the passage of substances from the gut into the bloodstream, triggering immune responses. This phenomenon, commonly referred to as leaky gut, has been linked to skin disorders, including eczema.

Inflammatory Mediators: Inflammatory molecules produced in the gut can circulate throughout the body and influence skin inflammation. Cytokines and other inflammatory mediators may contribute to the development and exacerbation of eczema.

Neuroendocrine Pathways: Communication between the gut and the skin also occurs through neuroendocrine pathways, involving the release of hormones and neurotransmitters. Stress, for example, can impact both the gut and the skin, exacerbating conditions like eczema (Aremu, 2021).

Understanding and addressing the gut-skin axis can help in the management and treatment of eczema. Strategies such as probiotic supplementation, dietary modifications, and lifestyle changes aimed at promoting a healthy gut environment may potentially alleviate eczema symptoms.

However, it's important to note that individual responses to these interventions may vary, and more research is needed to fully elucidate the complex relationship between the gut and skin in the context of eczema.

Psoriasis and Its Connection to Gut Inflammation

Psoriasis is a chronic autoimmune skin disorder characterized by the rapid buildup of skin cells, resulting in thick, red, and scaly patches on the skin. Although the precise cause of psoriasis is not fully understood, emerging evidence suggests a potential link between psoriasis and gut inflammation.

Several factors contribute to the connection between psoriasis and gut inflammation:

Immune System Dysregulation: Psoriasis is considered an immune-mediated disorder. Dysregulation of the immune system can lead to inflammation in various tissues, including the type of inflammation seen in the skin with psoriasis.

Gut Microbiota Imbalance: Studies have suggested that individuals with psoriasis may exhibit alterations in their gut microbiota that are not seen in those without the condition (Polak 2021).

Leaky Gut Syndrome: Some research indicates that individuals with psoriasis may experience higher levels of intestinal permeability (Sikora 2020).

Common Inflammatory Pathways: Psoriasis and inflammatory bowel diseases (IBD), such as Crohn's disease and ulcerative colitis, share some common inflammatory pathways. The inflammatory processes in the gut may influence systemic inflammation, affecting the skin and potentially contributing to the development or exacerbation of psoriasis.

Genetic Factors: Both psoriasis and certain gastrointestinal conditions have genetic components. Shared genetic susceptibility may contribute to the co-occurrence of psoriasis and gut inflammation in some individuals (Paul, 2022).

While the gut-skin axis and the link between psoriasis and gut inflammation are areas of ongoing research, it's important to note that not all individuals with psoriasis experience gastrointestinal issues, and the relationship can vary. Moreover, more research is needed to fully understand the mechanisms underlying this connection and to develop targeted therapeutic strategies.

Individuals with psoriasis may find that lifestyle and dietary changes, such as adopting an anti-inflammatory diet or taking probiotics, can have a positive impact on their skin condition.

However, individuals with psoriasis must consult with healthcare professionals for personalized advice and treatment options tailored to their specific needs.

Understanding the Connection between Gut Health and Aging Skin

Skin aging is a multifaceted process influenced by both intrinsic and extrinsic factors. While factors like sun exposure and genetics have long been recognized as key contributors to aging skin, emerging research suggests that the gut may also play a crucial role in this intricate balance.

Just like in previous discussions about the skin, the connection between gut health and skin aging revolves around the concept of the gut-skin axis. This relationship is mediated by various mechanisms that impact inflammation, nutrient absorption, and microbiota.

As we've seen, gut dysbiosis can trigger systemic inflammation, hastening the breakdown of skin collagen and elastin, ultimately contributing to the formation of wrinkles. Poor gut function may also lead to nutrient deficiencies, expediting the aging process of the skin.

Additionally, imbalances in the gut microbiota influence the immune system, contributing to the development of skin conditions such as acne and eczema, impacting overall skin health and aging.

The gut microbiota plays a role as well in its function of aiding in the regulation of hormones. Stress hormones compromise collagen production and accelerate skin aging.

Promoting gut health through dietary measures, incorporating probiotics, maintaining hydration, managing stress, and avoiding disruptive factors can positively influence skin aging.

Nutrients and Foods for Supporting Skin Elasticity and Preventing Aging

Here's a list of foods that are known to support skin elasticity:

- Fatty Fish: Salmon, mackerel, and other fatty fish are rich in omega-3 fatty acids, which help maintain skin cell membranes and contribute to overall skin health.

- Nuts and Seeds: Almonds, sunflower seeds, and walnuts provide vitamin E, which acts as an antioxidant and helps protect the skin from oxidative stress.

- Citrus Fruits: Oranges, lemons, and grapefruits are high in vitamin C, essential for collagen synthesis and promoting skin elasticity.

- Berries: Blueberries, strawberries, and raspberries are rich in antioxidants that combat free radicals and contribute to anti-aging effects.

- Avocado: This fruit is a good source of healthy fats, including monounsaturated fats, which can help maintain skin moisture and flexibility.

- Leafy Greens: Spinach, kale, and other leafy greens are packed with vitamins (like A, C, and E), minerals, and antioxidants that benefit skin health.

- Tomatoes: Tomatoes contain lycopene, a powerful antioxidant that may protect the skin from sun damage and contribute to skin elasticity.

- Sweet Potatoes: Rich in beta-carotene, sweet potatoes are converted into vitamin A in the body, promoting healthy skin and preventing signs of aging.

- Bell Peppers: Bell peppers, particularly red and yellow ones, are high in vitamin C and antioxidants that support collagen production.

- Broccoli: This vegetable is particularly rich in vitamins C and K, as well as antioxidants, contributing to overall skin health.

- Green Tea: Green tea contains polyphenols and antioxidants that may help protect the skin from aging and damage caused by free radicals.

- Watermelon: It not only hydrates but also contains lycopene and vitamins A and C, which are beneficial for the skin.

- Eggs: They provide essential amino acids and biotin, contributing to skin health and elasticity.

- Greek Yogurt: Greek yogurt is a good source of protein and probiotics, promoting overall skin health.

- Dark Chocolate: Because it contains flavonoids, it may contribute to skin hydration and protection against UV damage, if enjoyed in moderation.

Remember, maintaining a well-balanced and varied diet, staying hydrated, protecting your skin from excessive sun exposure, and adopting a healthy lifestyle are all crucial factors in supporting skin elasticity and preventing premature aging.

Nutrient-Rich Foods for Skin Health and Gut Nourishment

Consuming nutrient-rich foods is crucial for promoting both skin health and gut nourishment. The relationship between the gut and skin is evident, and a well-balanced diet can positively impact both areas. Below are nutrient-rich foods that contribute to skin health and support a thriving gut. By now, you should recognize a lot of these groups because they are ones that we've talked about in previous chapters. However, it's worth mentioning them again in the context of skin health, as the link between your skin and your gut is so strong.

Probiotic-Rich Foods:

- Yogurt: A natural source of probiotics, yogurt promotes a healthy gut microbiota, aiding digestion and supporting immune function.

- Kefir: This fermented dairy product contains probiotics and can contribute to a diverse and balanced gut microbiota.

Fiber-Rich Foods:

- Whole Grains: Foods like brown rice, quinoa, and oats provide fiber, promoting gut health by supporting the growth of beneficial bacteria.

- Legumes: Beans, lentils, and chickpeas are excellent sources of fiber, helping to maintain gut regularity and support a healthy microbiome.

Fruits and Vegetables:
- Berries: Rich in antioxidants, berries such as blueberries and strawberries help protect the skin from oxidative stress and inflammation.
- Leafy Greens: Spinach, kale, and Swiss chard are high in vitamins, minerals, and fiber, benefiting both gut health and skin radiance.

Fatty Fish:
- Salmon: A source of omega-3 fatty acids, salmon supports skin health by reducing inflammation and promoting skin hydration.

Nuts and Seeds:
- Almonds: Packed with vitamin E, almonds contribute to skin health by protecting against oxidative damage.
- Chia Seeds and Flaxseeds: High in omega-3 fatty acids and fiber, these seeds support gut health and have anti-inflammatory properties beneficial for the skin.

Protein Sources:
- Lean Poultry: Chicken and turkey provide protein necessary for skin repair and collagen synthesis.
- Plant-Based Proteins: Beans, lentils, tofu, and tempeh offer plant-based protein options that support both gut health and skin structure.

Fermented Foods:
- Sauerkraut: Fermented cabbage is rich in probiotics, promoting a healthy gut microbiota.

- Kimchi: A traditional Korean dish, it contains fermented vegetables and beneficial bacteria that contribute to gut health.

Colorful Vegetables:
- Carrots and Sweet Potatoes: Rich in beta-carotene, these vegetables contribute to skin health by supporting collagen production.

- Bell Peppers: High in vitamin C, bell peppers help in collagen synthesis and protect the skin from oxidative stress.

Tea:
- Green tea: Rich in antioxidants, green tea supports skin health by protecting against UV damage and promoting skin elasticity.

Water:
- Staying well-hydrated by drinking plenty of water is crucial for both gut health and skin hydration.

Incorporating a variety of these nutrient-rich foods into your diet supports a symbiotic relationship between gut health and skin vitality. A diverse and balanced diet nourishes the gut microbiota and provides essential nutrients that contribute to healthy, radiant skin.

Antioxidant-Rich Foods and the Benefits of Antioxidants

I'm going to focus on antioxidants in more detail here because they are so essential to the maintenance of skin health and gut nourishment. They do this through counteracting the harmful effects of free radicals in the body and unstable molecules that can cause cellular damage. Free radicals are produced through various processes, including exposure to UV rays, pollution, and normal metabolic activities.

Antioxidant-Rich Foods:

- Berries: Blueberries, strawberries, raspberries, and blackberries are packed with antioxidants like anthocyanins and vitamin C.

- Dark Leafy Greens: Spinach, kale, and Swiss chard contain antioxidants such as lutein, zeaxanthin, and beta-carotene.

- Nuts and Seeds: Almonds, walnuts, chia seeds, and flaxseeds provide vitamin E and other antioxidants.

- Fruits: Citrus fruits, like oranges and grapefruits, contain vitamin C, while avocados provide vitamin E.

- Colorful Vegetables: Carrots, sweet potatoes, and bell peppers are high in beta-carotene and other antioxidants.

- Green Tea: Rich in catechins, green tea has potent antioxidant properties.

- Spices: Turmeric, cinnamon, and ginger contain antioxidants and anti-inflammatory compounds.

- Dark Chocolate: High-quality dark chocolate is rich in flavonoids and can have antioxidant benefits (Jones, n.d.).

Incorporating a variety of antioxidant-rich foods into your diet can be fun. Plus, it brings a balanced and diverse diet for overall well-being.

Consulting with a healthcare professional or a nutritionist can provide personalized advice based on individual health needs.

Testimonials

"I struggled with persistent skin issues for years, battling everything from acne to dullness. Frustrated with conventional skincare remedies, I decided to focus on my gut health. After incorporating probiotic-rich foods and prebiotics into my diet, I noticed a remarkable change. My skin became clearer and more radiant, and the persistent redness faded away. The connection between gut health and skin vitality transformed not just my complexion but also my confidence." - **Julia Whiteman (41)**

"Eczema has been my constant companion since childhood. Tired of relying solely on topical treatments, I explored the link between gut health and skin conditions. By eliminating certain trigger foods and introducing gut-friendly options like fermented foods, I experienced a significant reduction in eczema flare-ups. It was a transformative journey that gave me not just relief from itching but also a newfound sense of control over my skin health." - **Alex Johnson (19)**

"My adult acne was not just a skin issue but a reflection of hormonal imbalance. Frustrated with antibiotics and harsh topical treatments, I decided to address the root cause. Through dietary changes, including hormone-balancing foods and supplements recommended by a nutritionist, I witnessed a gradual improvement. My skin became less prone to breakouts, and the painful cystic acne I once battled started to fade away. It was a reminder that, sometimes, the most effective solutions come from within." - **Camille Thompson (25)**

"As I approached my forties, signs of aging began affecting my skin. Intrigued by the gut-skin connection, I revamped my diet with collagen-rich foods and gut-supporting nutrients. Over time, not only did my skin regain elasticity, but fine lines also seemed to diminish. I felt like I had turned back the clock, showcasing that nourishing the gut could indeed be a natural fountain of youth for the skin." - **Dan Seth (43)**

Creating a personalized approach to improving gut health for better skin quality involves a combination of dietary, lifestyle, and wellness strategies. Below is a planning tool that you can use to guide the process:

1. Evaluation

Assessment of Gut Health: Evaluate current gut health by examining symptoms and consider professional testing if necessary.

Skin Evaluation: Assess the current state of the skin, noting any issues such as acne or inflammation.

2. Goal Setting

Establish Clear Objectives: Set specific and measurable goals for both gut health and skin improvement.

Timeline Planning: Define a realistic timeline for achieving these goals.

3. Dietary Adjustments

Incorporate Gut-Boosting Foods: Integrate probiotic-rich and prebiotic-rich foods to enhance the gut microbiome.

Hydration Focus: Ensure sufficient water intake to support digestion and skin hydration.

Explore Elimination Diet: Identify and remove potential food triggers through an elimination diet.

4. Supplementation

Probiotic Inclusion: Introduce a quality probiotic supplement to support a healthy gut.

Omega-3 Fatty Acids: Consider adding omega-3 supplements to reduce inflammation and promote skin health.

Collagen Boost: Incorporate collagen supplements to enhance skin elasticity.

5. Lifestyle Modifications

Regular Exercise: Include consistent physical activity to support overall well-being and skin health.

Stress Management Techniques: Implement stress-reducing practices like meditation, yoga, or deep breathing.

Prioritize Adequate Sleep: Ensure 7 to 9 hours of quality sleep to facilitate skin regeneration.

6. Skincare Routine

Gentle Cleansing: Opt for a mild, non-stripping cleanser suitable for your skin type.

Hydration Practices: Use a hydrating moisturizer to maintain skin moisture.

Sun Protection: Apply sunscreen with sufficient SPF to shield the skin from harmful UV rays.

7. Monitoring and Adjustments

Maintain a Journal: Keep a journal to track food intake and symptoms for progress assessment.

Regular Check-Ins: Schedule periodic check-ins to evaluate changes in gut health and skin condition.

Flexibility for Adjustments: Modify the plan based on feedback from your body and progress toward your goals.

8. Professional Guidance

Consult with Experts: Seek advice from a registered dietitian, dermatologist, or healthcare professional for personalized guidance.

Routine Health Check-ups: Schedule regular health check-ups to monitor overall well-being.

Consistency and patience are crucial for success, and adjustments may be necessary as your body responds to the changes. Always consult with healthcare professionals before making significant dietary or lifestyle changes, especially if you have pre-existing health conditions.

CHAPTER EIGHT

Digestive Health through Life's Stages

We will now explore the dynamic connection between digestive health and the various stages of life. From early childhood to the golden years of aging, our digestive systems undergo significant transformations that profoundly impact our overall well-being.

Did you know that, according to research, from infancy, the choices made regarding early feeding practices can significantly impact gut health? The composition of the gut microbiome is particularly influenced by factors such as the types of foods introduced early on and the methods of feeding.

These early influences play a crucial role in shaping a healthy and diverse gut microbiota in infants, with potential long-term effects on digestive health and overall well-being throughout various life stages. Recognizing the importance of these early choices is essential for fostering a resilient and balanced gut microbiome right from the earliest stages of life.

Nurturing a Healthy Gut from Birth

Promoting gut health in childhood is crucial for overall well-being, as the early years establish the foundation for a resilient digestive system. Nurturing a healthy gut from birth is particularly important, as it can have lasting effects on a child's health and development. As we explore the wonders of gut health, know that every feeding choice contributes to your child's well-being and embrace the unique journey you've chosen for your little one. Here are key considerations in understanding and supporting gut health in childhood:

Microbial Colonization at Birth:

The process of microbial colonization begins at birth, where a newborn's gut is populated by microorganisms from the mother, the environment, and the delivery method. Vaginal births expose infants to the mother's microbiota, while cesarean births may result in a different microbial composition. Take comfort in knowing that both paths, although different, play a crucial role in establishing a diverse and resilient gut microbiome.

The Role of Breastfeeding:

Breastfeeding also contributes significantly to the establishment of a diverse and beneficial gut microbiome. Breast milk is rich in nutrients and bioactive compounds that support the growth of beneficial bacteria in the infant's gut. It contains prebiotics, probiotics, and antibodies that contribute to the development of a robust immune system and a healthy gut microbiome. Breastfeeding is recognized for its role in reducing the risk of various digestive issues and promoting optimal gut health in early childhood. While breastfeeding has its unique benefits, formula feeding comes with its own set of nurturing moments. Although breast milk is a powerhouse of nutrients and bioactive compounds, formula feeding also provides a reliable source of nutrition tailored to your baby's needs.

Introduction of Solid Foods:

As a child transitions to solid foods, a diverse diet becomes crucial for nurturing a healthy gut. Introducing a variety of fruits, vegetables, whole grains, and other nutrient-rich foods supports the growth of a diverse microbial community. Avoiding excessive use of antibiotics and processed foods is also essential, as these factors can disrupt the balance of gut bacteria.

Importance of Fiber:

Dietary fiber plays a key role in promoting gut health by acting as a prebiotic, providing fuel for beneficial bacteria. Including fiber-rich foods in a child's diet, such as fruits, vegetables, and whole grains, helps maintain a healthy balance of gut microbiota, aiding in digestion and nutrient absorption.

Proactive Health Measures:

Ensuring good hygiene practices, promoting physical activity, and encouraging healthy sleeping patterns are proactive measures that contribute to maintaining a healthy gut in childhood. These practices help preserve the delicate balance of the gut microbiome and support the development of a robust immune system.

Birth Methods and Gut Considerations

An impacted gut can lead to colic and congestion.

An impacted gut in babies can lead to colic and congestion, due to factors like constipation, gut microbiome imbalance, feeding issues, and reflux. Constipation causes abdominal discomfort and contributes to colic, while an imbalanced gut microbiome can result in gas and digestive discomfort. Introducing new formulas or sudden dietary changes may also impact the gut. Gastroesophageal reflux (GERD) associated with an impacted gut can cause congestion and respiratory issues. Probiotics, dietary adjustments, and maintaining hydration are strategies to address and prevent these issues.

C-section babies will need early prebiotic and probiotic support.

C-section babies, those delivered through cesarean section, can benefit from early pre and probiotic support to encourage optimal gut health. Unlike infants born through natural delivery, C-section babies do not have the opportunity to be exposed to their mother's vaginal and fecal microbes, which are essential for seeding their gut with beneficial bacteria.

- *Absence of Vaginal Microbial Transfer:* C-section births lack exposure to the beneficial microbes found in the birth canal, potentially affecting the initial composition of the infant's gut microbiota.

- *Significance of Early Microbial Colonization:* Early microbial colonization is crucial for developing a diverse and balanced gut microbiome, influencing various aspects of health such as immune function, metabolism, and digestion.

- *Probiotics for C-section Babies:* Administering probiotics, live beneficial bacteria, may help establish a healthy gut microbiome in C-section babies. Commonly used probiotic strains for infants include Lactobacillus and Bifidobacterium.

- *Prebiotics to Support Probiotics:* The introduction of prebiotics—non-digestible fibers promoting the growth of beneficial bacteria—can support the effectiveness of probiotics.

- *Potential Health Benefits:* Early pre and probiotic supplementation in C-section babies could potentially reduce the risk of conditions such as allergies, asthma, and other immune-related disorders. Improved gut health may contribute to better nutrient absorption and overall well-being.

- *Breastfeeding as a Natural Source:* Breast milk itself contains beneficial microbes and serves as a natural source of prebiotics, supporting the establishment of a healthy gut microbiome in infants.

- *Formula feeding as an Alternative:* Formula brings its own set of nurturing moments, offering a dependable source of nutrition that is customized to meet your baby's requirements.

All in all, while additional research is necessary, early pre and probiotic support for C-section babies may help compensate for the lack of natural microbial exposure during birth.

Parent Testimonials

"I observed a fascinating connection between my child's mood and digestive health. When we incorporated probiotic-rich foods into their diet, they seemed happier and more content. It was a personal realization of the potential link between early gut health and the development of a positive mood in infants." - **Emily & Patrick**

"Dealing with an infant suffering from reflux was challenging. After consulting with a healthcare professional, we introduced probiotics into our baby's routine, leading to a noticeable reduction in reflux symptoms." - **Jane & Isaac**

"Having children born through both C-section and natural births, we noticed distinct differences in their gut health. Our child born through natural birth appeared to have a more robust digestive system and experienced fewer tummy troubles." - **Ilena & Jack**

"We faced the challenging period of dealing with a colicky baby. It was tough to see our little one in distress. After consulting with our healthcare professional, we decided to try probiotics. Gradually, we noticed a reduction in colic symptoms, and our baby seemed more at ease." - **Kate & Mark**

Further Strategies to Support Gut Health in Newborns and Babies

- *Fiber for Moms*: Maintain a diet rich in fiber during pregnancy by incorporating fruits, grains, nuts, legumes, and vegetables.

- *Delayed First Bath*: Postponing the first bath provides multiple benefits, including enhanced bonding and protection against infections.

Probiotics for Moms: Mothers can consider prenatal probiotics for potential benefits.

A Young Girl's Journey through Intestinal Challenges

Mia's story unfolded in a small town, where she faced the unique challenge of gastroschisis. Born with her intestines outside her tiny body, Mia found solace at Lucile Packard Children's Hospital at Stanford. Lily, her adoptive mother, became a pillar of strength in navigating the complexities of intestinal failure and total parenteral nutrition (TPN) dependence during Mia's early years.

The gradual transformation in Mia's life was marked by the delicate dance of medical care and Lily's unwavering dedication. Specialists at the hospital guided caring for Mia, ensuring her nutritional needs were met through personalized plans.

Mia's journey toward independence from TPN was a remarkable testament to adaptation. She now joyfully partakes in family meals from minimal food intake as a toddler. Regular checkups, orchestrated by a dedicated healthcare team, fine-tune Mia's nutrition plan, ensuring her growth and well-being.

Lily's goal mirrored the determination of many caregivers—to guide Mia toward independence from TPN. The support Mia found in her journey through personalized eating plans, enhanced by a tenacious spirit, ensured her success. Today, Mia, a spirited eight-year-old, thrives with reduced TPN support, embodying resilience and triumph (Nichols, 2020).

Exploring Dietary Habits for Optimal Gut Health in Kids

Here are some tips on how you can improve gut health in your children:

- Emphasize breastfeeding during the initial six months and continue as long as possible to establish a healthy gut flora.

- Maintain a balanced diet with a variety of soluble and insoluble fiber-rich foods like quinoa, oats, lentils, and beans.

- Limit the intake of fatty foods, junk food, caffeinated beverages, and candy. Instead, focus on incorporating healthy fats and high-fiber foods for optimal digestion.

- Include easily digestible lean meats, such as chicken, to support improved digestion and nutrient absorption.

- Integrate probiotics into their diet through natural sources, like yogurt, kefir, and sauerkraut, or consider a pediatrician-recommended probiotic supplement.

- Choose small, frequent meals to facilitate easier consumption, provide sustained energy, and maintain continuous digestive system activity.

- Ensure proper hydration with water or alternatives like fruit-infused water, fresh fruit juices, tender coconut water, melons, and cucumbers.

- Encourage regular physical activity, including exercises and specific yoga poses, to promote overall well-being and stimulate the digestive system.

- Use antibiotics judiciously, avoiding unnecessary courses to preserve long-term gut health.

- Promote outdoor exposure to germs for enhanced gut and immune health, emphasizing basic hygiene without over-sanitizing to build natural immunity (*10 Tips to Maintain a Healthy Gut in Kids*, n.d.).

Common Digestive Challenges in Children and How to Address Them

Children may encounter a range of digestive challenges, including issues like constipation, diarrhea, GERD, food allergies, IBS, lactose intolerance, celiac disease, bloating, gas, and overeating.

Managing these concerns often involves dietary adjustments, such as ensuring sufficient fiber intake and avoiding trigger foods. Lifestyle factors, including hydration, regular physical activity, and consistent routines, are crucial for digestive health.

Additionally, seeking guidance from healthcare professionals is vital for accurate diagnosis and personalized management plans tailored to the child's needs. Encouraging mindful eating habits and providing a balanced diet contribute to overall digestive well-being, supporting a healthy foundation for children's growth and development.

Women, Hormones, and Gut Changes: Why Your Gut Gets Worse during Your Cycle

Women undergo natural hormonal fluctuations during their menstrual cycle, mainly involving estrogen and progesterone. These changes can influence digestive function. In the first half of the cycle, estrogen levels rise, peaking before ovulation, while the second half sees increased progesterone to prepare for potential pregnancy. These hormonal shifts can affect the gut in various ways:

- *Slowed Digestion:* Elevated progesterone relaxes smooth muscle tissue, including the digestive tract muscles, leading to slower transit times and feelings of bloating or constipation.

- *Water Retention:* Hormonal changes may disturb water balance, causing some women to experience bloating and discomfort due to water retention.

- *Sensitivity to Pain:* Hormones influence pain perception, potentially making some women more sensitive to abdominal discomfort or cramping during their menstrual period.

- *Microbiome Changes:* Hormonal fluctuations can impact the gut microbiome, affecting the composition and activity of microorganisms in the digestive tract. This can potentially lead to gut symptoms that include digestive discomfort, irregular bowel movements, increased food sensitivity, anxiety, stress, or mood swings.

- *Increased Sensitivity:* Some women may experience heightened gut sensitivity during their menstrual cycle, resulting in increased discomfort or symptoms associated with conditions like irritable bowel syndrome (IBS) (*Gut Health and Your Menstrual Cycle: What Women Need to Know*, 2022).

Individual responses to these changes vary. While some women may not notice significant digestive alterations, others may experience pronounced symptoms.

Managing these effects involves maintaining a healthy diet, staying hydrated, engaging in regular physical activity, and considering stress reduction techniques. Dietary adjustments and lifestyle modifications can often alleviate symptoms associated with hormonal fluctuations, promoting better digestive health.

Seniors Experiencing Improved Quality of Life Through Gut Health Support

"Seeking a solution to my digestive issues, I consulted with a nutritionist who recommended focusing on gut health. I adjusted my diet, incorporating more fiber-rich foods and probiotics. As time passed, I noticed a remarkable improvement in my digestion, with reduced discomfort and increased energy levels. Now, I happily share my personal success story, emphasizing the transformative impact of prioritizing gut health on my overall well-being." - **Elsa (75)**

"I embraced a holistic approach to gut health with guidance from my healthcare provider. By introducing fermented foods and prebiotics into my diet, I experienced gradual but significant positive changes. My digestive issues subsided, and I discovered a renewed sense of well-being. Now, I encourage others in my age group to prioritize gut health, believing it's never too late to embark on a journey toward improved vitality." - **James (68)**

Understanding Changes in the Gut as We Age

As we age, several changes occur in the gut. Muscle strength and coordination decline, leading to slower digestion and potential constipation. Digestive enzyme production also decreases, which in turn affects nutrient absorption. In addition to this, the gut microbiome undergoes alterations, and the intestinal lining may thin, making the gut more susceptible to irritation. Plus, stomach acid production decreases, impacting nutrient absorption. The risk of gastrointestinal disorders, like diverticulosis and IBS, also increases with age.

To support gut health, maintain a balanced diet that includes plenty of fiber, stay hydrated, exercise regularly, consider probiotics, and undergo regular health check-ups for early detection and management of digestive conditions.

Nutrition for Healthy Aging

"At seventy-two, I faced digestive discomfort affecting my daily life. After consulting a nutritionist, I embraced a gut-friendly diet rich in fiber, fruits, and probiotics. The change was remarkable. Gradually, my digestive issues eased, and I regained vitality. Now, at seventy-five, I enjoy each day with newfound comfort, all thanks to prioritizing my gut health through simple dietary changes." - **Clara**

"In my late sixties, digestive challenges made me apprehensive about enjoying my golden years. With guidance from a healthcare professional, I adopted a balanced diet with whole grains and fermented foods. The impact on my gut health was significant—less bloating, improved regularity, and increased energy. Now, at seventy-two, I savor life's moments with a renewed sense of well-being, grateful for the positive changes a gut-friendly diet brought to my daily life." - **Vivien**

Dietary Recommendations for Maintaining Gut Health in the Elderly

Maintaining gut health is crucial for individuals aged fifty and above due to changes in the digestive system with age. Here are specific dietary recommendations tailored for older adults:

- *Fiber-Rich Foods:* Prioritize a diet high in fiber from sources like whole grains, fruits, vegetables, and legumes to prevent constipation and support digestive health.

- *Probiotics and Fermented Foods:* Include probiotic-rich foods, such as yogurt, kefir, sauerkraut, and kimchi, to introduce beneficial bacteria to the gut, aiding in digestion and helping to maintain a balanced microbiome.

- *Adequate Hydration:* Ensure sufficient water intake throughout the day to support the mucous layer in the intestines, preventing constipation and promoting overall digestive well-being.

- *Prebiotic-Rich Foods:* Incorporate prebiotic foods, like garlic, onions, bananas, and asparagus, into meals to act as fuel for beneficial gut bacteria, promoting their growth and activity.

- *Lean Proteins:* Choose lean protein sources, such as poultry, fish, and plant-based proteins, which are easier on the digestive system and contribute to overall gut health.

- *Whole Grains:* Choose whole grains like brown rice, quinoa, and whole wheat for their fiber and nutrient content, supporting digestive health and regularity.

- *Limit Processed Foods:* Reduce the consumption of processed foods, focusing on whole, minimally processed options to avoid additives that can disrupt the balance of the gut microbiome.

- *Moderate Fat Intake:* Maintain a balanced intake of healthy fats from sources like olive oil, avocados, and nuts to support nutrient absorption and contribute to overall gut function.

- *Diverse Diet:* Aim for a diverse and well-balanced diet, including a variety of fruits, vegetables, whole grains, and proteins to promote a diverse microbiome crucial for gut health.

- *Consult with a Healthcare Professional:* Given that individual dietary needs can vary, older adults should consult healthcare professionals or registered dietitians for personalized recommendations, considering specific health conditions, medications, and dietary preferences.

- *Monitor Lactose Intake:* Be mindful of lactose intolerance that may develop with age, monitor dairy intake, and consider lactose-free alternatives if necessary (*Nutrition Needs When You're Over 65*, n.d.).

By incorporating these age-specific dietary recommendations, individuals aged fifty and above can actively promote their gut health, enhance digestive function, and contribute to overall well-being. It's advisable to approach dietary changes gradually and seek professional guidance for personalized advice tailored to individual health needs.

This chapter focused on how our gut, like any other organ, can behave differently at every stage of our life. From childhood to our older years, the way our gut behaves can change. Next up is the epilogue, where you can find encouragement from some amazing success stories.

Real Stories of Gut Transformation

"I battled persistent bloating and irregular bowel habits that significantly impacted my daily life. Consulting with a healthcare professional, I discovered an imbalanced gut microbiome. Taking charge of my gut health, I adopted a diet rich in fiber, probiotics, and prebiotics. Gradually, my symptoms were alleviated, and I restored balance to my digestion. Today, I maintain my gut health with a diverse and wholesome diet." - **Olivia (55)**

"I faced ongoing indigestion and discomfort following meals. A thorough examination revealed reduced stomach acid production as the root cause. Making dietary adjustments, I opted for smaller, more frequent meals and introduced digestive enzymes. This approach proved successful as my symptoms improved, allowing me to savor meals without prior discomfort." - **James (60)**

"I confronted challenges with constipation and sluggish digestion. Identifying a deficiency in dietary fiber, I revamped my eating habits, embracing whole grains, fruits, and vegetables. This dietary shift notably enhanced my bowel regularity, underscoring the significance of a fiber-rich diet for gut health."- **Sophie (27)**

"I experienced recurring digestive upset and bloating, attributing it to an imbalance in my gut microbiome. Taking proactive steps, I incorporated probiotic-rich foods and supplements into my daily routine. Over time, my gut balance was restored, and I found relief from digestive discomfort." - **Nathan (32)**

"I dealt with intermittent constipation and low energy levels. Identifying inadequate hydration as a contributing factor, I prioritized water intake, especially during meals. This simple adjustment resulted in improved digestion, heightened energy, and an overall sense of well-being. My commitment to hydration became a cornerstone for maintaining my gut health." - **Anna (41)**

Conclusion

We are now wrapping up our exploration of digestive health. We've delved into various aspects, from understanding digestion and unraveling digestive disorders to exploring the gut-brain connection and making informed lifestyle choices for digestive wellness. Our journey has covered healing herbs, the impact of gut health on skin and immunity, and considerations for digestive well-being through different life stages. The epilogue serves as a testament to the practical application of the insights provided throughout this book.

The central message resounds clearly: the well-being of our gut profoundly influences our overall health. The crux of our journey is the importance of nurturing and maintaining a healthy gut for a thriving life. It goes beyond mere dietary choices; it encompasses the profound impact that such choices have on our physical, mental, and emotional health.

The three real-life stories shared in the introduction illustrated the widespread challenges faced by individuals neglecting their gut health.

Sandra, Jenny, and Claire encountered various health issues, underscoring the far-reaching consequences of an unhealthy gut.

Returning to these stories, we witnessed the transformative power of knowledge and intentional choices. Sandra found balance in her hectic life by prioritizing nourishing foods and managing stress. Jenny regained vitality, overcoming stomach issues and restoring her well-being through mindful dietary changes. Claire, a professional with a demanding lifestyle, took control of her health through balanced meals and physical activity.

These success stories highlight a fundamental truth: every small choice impacts our gut and, consequently, our future health and well-being. Change, no matter how small, can lead to significant transformations. The journey toward a healthier gut begins with the smallest, easiest steps. The very first? A commitment to making mindful choices today.

As you embark on your journey to digestive wellness, remember the lessons learned within these pages. Embrace the power of informed decisions, mindful nourishment, and the remarkable connection between your gut and overall health. Your gut is not just a digestive organ; it's a cornerstone of your well-being.

Consider this a call to action: Start today, armed with newfound knowledge and inspired by the success stories within! Your gut transformation awaits, and your future self will undoubtedly thank you for this investment in your health. If this journey has resonated with you, share your thoughts and experiences. Your genuine reflections may inspire others to take the first step toward a healthier digestive system. Here's to your journey into a vibrant, gut-healthy life!

Share the Knowledge

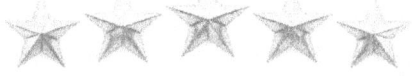

Now that you have all the tools to embark on your gut-healing journey, it's time to pay it forward and guide other readers to the same transformative knowledge.

By sharing your honest thoughts about this book on Amazon, you're not just leaving a review; you're illuminating the path for fellow readers. Your review becomes a compass, directing others to the information they seek and fostering their passion for understanding leaky gut and digestive health.

Your contribution is priceless. The passion for self-education and understanding thrives when we share our newfound knowledge—and you're playing a pivotal role in making that happen.

Click Here to leave your review on Amazon.

Thank you for being an integral part of this mission. The journey of self-education and understanding continues when we generously share our insights with others.

With gratitude,

Dr. Ashley Sullivan, PharmD, RPh, MBA

Ways to Connect:

Follow Dr. Ashley Sullivan, PharmD on Facebook, link below

https://www.facebook.com/profile.php?id=100092716005488

Website

Join her FREE Facebook group "Compassionate Care and Holistic Advocacy with Dr. Ashley", link below.

https://www.facebook.com/groups/907620087038942

Gut Friendly Recipes

Quinoa Parfait

Ingredients:
- ½ cup cooked quinoa
- ½ cup Greek yogurt
- 1 tablespoon honey
- ¼ cup fresh berries (blueberries, strawberries, or raspberries)
- 1 tablespoon chia seeds
- 1 tablespoon chopped nuts (almonds, walnuts, or pistachios)

Instructions:
- In a bowl, layer half of the cooked quinoa.
- Add a layer of Greek yogurt on top of the quinoa.

- Drizzle honey over the yogurt layer.
- Sprinkle fresh berries evenly over the honey layer.
- Add the remaining quinoa on top of the berries.
- Sprinkle chia seeds and chopped nuts over the final quinoa layer.
- Serve chilled and enjoy this nutritious and gut-supportive breakfast parfait.

Grilled Salmon with Quinoa and Roasted Vegetables

Ingredients:
- 1 salmon fillet
- 1 cup cooked quinoa
- 1 cup mixed vegetables (bell peppers, zucchini, cherry tomatoes)
- 1 tablespoon olive oil
- 1 teaspoon lemon juice
- Salt and pepper to taste
- Fresh herbs for garnish (parsley or dill)

Instructions:
- Preheat the grill or oven to medium-high heat.
- Season the salmon fillet with salt, pepper, and lemon juice.
- In a bowl, toss the mixed vegetables with olive oil, salt, and

pepper.

- Grill or roast the salmon fillet and mixed vegetables until cooked through.

- Place a serving of cooked quinoa on a plate.

- Top with grilled salmon and roasted vegetables.

- Garnish with fresh herbs.

- Serve warm and savor this satisfying and digestion-friendly main course.

Ginger Turmeric Tea

Ingredients:

- 1-inch piece of fresh ginger, sliced

- 1 teaspoon ground turmeric

- 1 tablespoon honey

- 1 lemon wedge

- 2 cups hot water

Instructions:

- In a teapot, combine ginger slices, ground turmeric, and honey.

- Squeeze the lemon wedge into the mixture.

- Pour hot water over the ingredients.

- Let it steep for 5-7 minutes.

- Strain the tea into a cup.
- Enjoy this soothing and gut-supportive beverage for a refreshing snack.

Probiotic-Rich Smoothie

Ingredients:
- 1 cup Greek yogurt
- 1 ripe banana
- 1/2 cup mixed berries (blueberries, strawberries, or raspberries)
- 1 tablespoon honey
- 1/2 cup kefir

Directions:
- Place all ingredients in a blender.
- Blend until smooth.
- Pour into a glass and enjoy your probiotic-rich smoothie!

Quinoa Salad with Fermented Veggies

Ingredients:
- 1 cup cooked quinoa
- 1/2 cup fermented vegetables (kimchi, sauerkraut)
- 1 cucumber, diced
- Lemon-tahini dressing (1 tablespoon tahini, juice of 1 lemon, salt)

Directions:

- In a bowl, combine quinoa, fermented veggies, and diced cucumber.

- In a small bowl, whisk together the lemon-tahini dressing.

- Pour the dressing over the quinoa mixture and toss to combine.

Ginger Turmeric Carrot Soup

Ingredients:

- 4 cups carrots, chopped

- 1 tablespoon fresh ginger, grated

- 1 tablespoon fresh turmeric, grated

- 4 cups vegetable broth

- 1 cup coconut milk

- Salt and black pepper to taste

Directions:

- In a pot, combine carrots, ginger, turmeric, and vegetable broth.

- Bring to a boil, then simmer until carrots are tender.

- Blend the mixture until smooth, then return to the pot.

- Stir in coconut milk and season with salt and pepper.

Salmon and Avocado Salad:

Ingredients:

- 2 cups mixed greens
- 6 oz grilled salmon, flaked
- 1 avocado, sliced
- Cherry tomatoes, halved
- Olive oil and lemon dressing

Directions:
- Arrange mixed greens on a plate.
- Top with grilled salmon, avocado slices, and cherry tomatoes.
- Drizzle with olive oil and lemon dressing.

Chickpea and Vegetable Stir-Fry
Ingredients:
- 1 can chickpeas, drained and rinsed
- Mixed vegetables (bell peppers, broccoli, snap peas)
- 2 cloves garlic, minced
- 2 tablespoons tamari or soy sauce
- 1 tablespoon sesame oil

Directions:
- In a pan, sauté garlic in sesame oil.
- Add mixed vegetables and chickpeas, stir-fry until tender.
- Pour tamari or soy sauce, toss until well-coated.

Blueberry Chia Pudding

Ingredients:

- 1/4 cup chia seeds
- 1 cup almond milk
- 1/2 cup blueberries (fresh or frozen)
- 1 tablespoon honey
- Almonds for topping

Directions:

- In a jar, mix chia seeds and almond milk. Refrigerate for a few hours or overnight.
- Layer with blueberries and drizzle honey.
- Top with almonds before serving.

Roasted Turmeric Cauliflower

Ingredients:

- 1 head cauliflower, cut into florets
- 2 tablespoons olive oil
- 1 teaspoon turmeric
- 1/2 teaspoon cumin
- Salt and pepper to taste

Directions:

- Toss cauliflower in olive oil, turmeric, cumin, salt, and pepper.

- Roast in the oven until golden brown.

Gut-Healing Green Smoothie

Ingredients:
- 1 cup kale or spinach
- 1/2 cucumber
- 1/2 banana
- 1/2 cup pineapple chunks
- 1 cup coconut water

Directions:
- Blend all ingredients until smooth.
- Pour into a glass and enjoy your green smoothie.

Feel free to adjust the quantities and ingredients based on your preferences and dietary needs. These recipes aim to provide nourishment and support for a healthy gut!

Medications for Digestive Disorders

Embarking on a journey toward optimal gut health involves a comprehensive approach, with lifestyle playing a pivotal role. My primary focus is to uncover and address the root causes of digestive issues, promoting holistic well-being. However, I recognize that symptoms can sometimes disrupt your daily life and well-being, necessitating additional support. As a pharmacist, this book wouldn't be complete without discussing all the options.

In this section, I provide valuable insights into medications commonly used to address digestive concerns. It's essential to approach medication as a complementary tool alongside lifestyle changes, aiming for a balanced and personalized approach to enhance your digestive wellness. Let's explore the medications frequently employed in the realm of digestive health, understanding their roles and how they can contribute to your journey toward a healthier gut.

Antacids:

- Examples include calcium carbonate (found in Tums) and a combination of aluminum hydroxide/magnesium hydroxide (Maalox). Other options are Pepto-Bismol, Rolaids, and Mylanta.

- These medications alleviate symptoms of heartburn and indigestion by neutralizing excess stomach acid.

Proton Pump Inhibitors (PPIs):
- Examples of PPIs are Omeprazole (sold as Prilosec), Esomeprazole (Nexium), and Lansoprazole (Prevacid). Other brands include Protonix, Aciphex, and Dexilant.

- PPIs are used for the short-term treatment of gastroesophageal reflux disease (GERD) and peptic ulcers, as they reduce the production of stomach acid.

H2 Blockers (Histamine-2 Receptor Antagonists):
- Examples of H2 blockers are Ranitidine (Zantac), Famotidine (Pepcid), and Cimetidine (Tagamet).

- These medications relieve symptoms of heartburn and indigestion by blocking histamine, which in turn reduces the production of stomach acid.

Antispasmodics:
- Examples of antispasmodics include Dicyclomine (Bentyl) and Hyoscyamine (Levsin).

- These medications help alleviate abdominal cramps and spasms by relaxing the smooth muscles in the digestive tract.

Laxatives:

- Examples of laxatives include Psyllium (Metamucil), Bisacodyl (Dulcolax), Polyethylene Glycol (Miralax), and Senokot.

- These medications relieve constipation by promoting bowel movements.

Antidiarrheals:
- Examples include Loperamide (Imodium) and Bismuth Subsalicylate (found in Pepto-Bismol).

- They are used to slow down bowel movements and reduce inflammation, providing relief from diarrhea.

Antiemetics (for nausea and vomiting):
- Examples are Ondansetron (Zofran), Metoclopramide (Reglan), and Dimenhydrinate (Dramamine).

- These medications suppress nausea and vomiting.

Stool Softeners:
- Docusate (Colace) is often used.

- This medication relieves difficulty passing stools by adding moisture to them, making them easier to pass.

Prokinetic Agents (to improve gastrointestinal motility):
- Examples include Metoclopramide (Reglan) and Domperidone.

- These medications enhance gastrointestinal motility.

Digestive Enzymes:
- Examples include Pancrelipase (Creon, Pancreaze) and Lac-

tase supplements (Lactaid).

- These medications aid in the digestion of nutrients and are used for digestive enzyme deficiencies.

Antiflatulents:
- Examples include Simethicone (Gas-X) and Charcoal (activated charcoal).

- These medications break down gas bubbles, providing relief from gas and bloating.

Gastrointestinal Protective Agents:
- An example is Sucralfate (Carafate).

- This medication forms a protective barrier on the stomach lining, providing relief from peptic ulcers and gastritis.

Hepatoprotective Agents (for liver health):
- Examples include Ursodiol (Actigall) and Silymarin (Milk Thistle).

- These medications support and protect liver function.

Antiulcer Agents (for preventing and treating ulcers):
- Examples include Misoprostol (Cytotec) and Rebamipide (Mucosta).

- These medications promote healing and reduce the formation of peptic ulcers.

Gallstone Dissolving Agents:
- An example is Ursodiol (Actigall).

- This medication is used to dissolve cholesterol-based gallstones.

Bile Acid Sequestrants (for cholesterol management):
- Examples include Cholestyramine (Questran) and Colesevelam (Welchol).

- These medications reduce cholesterol absorption by binding to bile acids.

Anti-inflammatory Agents (for inflammatory bowel diseases):
- Examples include Mesalamine (Asacol, Pentasa) and Prednisone.

- These medications reduce inflammation in the digestive tract, providing relief from inflammatory bowel diseases.

Antibiotics (for bacterial infections in the GI tract):
- Examples include Ciprofloxacin (Cipro) and Metronidazole (Flagyl).

- These medications are used to treat bacterial infections in the gastrointestinal tract.

Immunosuppressants (for autoimmune conditions of the digestive system):
- Examples include Azathioprine (Imuran) and Infliximab (Remicade).

- These medications suppress the immune response and are used to treat autoimmune conditions affecting the digestive system.

Opioid Receptor Antagonists (for opioid-induced constipation):
- Examples include Naloxegol (Movantik) and Methylnaltrexone (Relistor).

- These medications block the constipating effects of opioids and provide relief from constipation caused by opioid use.

Suspected Gut-Unfriendly Medications

The following list of medications are often suspected to have potential effects on gut health based on common knowledge. Please note that individual reactions may vary, and it's important to consult with a healthcare professional for personalized advice. Here are some medications that are often discussed in relation to potential impacts on gut health:

- Antibiotics: They can disrupt the balance of gut bacteria by killing both harmful and beneficial microbes.

- Non-Steroidal Anti-Inflammatory Drugs (NSAIDs): Regular use of NSAIDs, such as ibuprofen and aspirin, may lead to irritation and damage to the gastrointestinal tract.

- Proton Pump Inhibitors (PPIs): These drugs reduce stomach acid production and may affect the balance of gut bacteria.

- Steroids: Long-term use of corticosteroids can impact the gut microbiota.

- Birth Control Pills: Hormonal contraceptives may influence gut health in some individuals.

- Antidepressants: Some antidepressants may have effects on the gut microbiota.

- Immunosuppressants: Medications that suppress the immune system may have an impact on gut health.

It's important to emphasize that the impact of medications on gut health can vary from person to person, and in many cases, the benefits of these medications may outweigh any potential negative effects on gut health. If you have concerns about the medications, you are taking and their impact on your gut health, it's best to discuss them with your healthcare provider. They can provide personalized advice based on your specific health needs and conditions.

References

1. Anguita-Ruiz A, Aguilera CM, Gil Á. Genetics of Lactose Intolerance: An Updated Review and Online Interactive World Maps of Phenotype and Genotype Frequencies. Nutrients. 2020 Sep 3;12(9):2689. doi: 10.3390/nu12092689. PMID: 32899182; PMCID: PMC7551416.

2. Appleton J. (2018). The Gut-Brain Axis: Influence of Microbiota on Mood and Mental Health. Integrative medicine (Encinitas, Calif.), 17(4), 28–32.

3. Appleton J. (2018). The Gut-Brain Axis: Influence of Microbiota on Mood and Mental Health. *Integrative medicine (Encinitas, Calif.), 17*(4), 28–32.

4. Barbara Bolen, P. (2022, September 6). *Why enzymes are an important part of your digestive system*. Verywell Health. https://www.verywellhealth.com/what-are-digestive-enzymes-1945036

5. Barbara Bolen, P. (2022a, September 6). *Why enzymes are an important part of your digestive system.* Verywell Health. https://www.verywellhealth.com/what-are-digestive-enzymes-1945036

6. Case-Lo, C. (2020, November 5). *How does serotonin in the brain affect your bowels?.* Healthline. https://www.healthline.com/health/irritable-bowel-syndrome/serotonin-effects

7. *Constipation symptoms and treatments.* NHS inform. (1BC, November 30). https://www.nhsinform.scot/illnesses-and-conditions/stomach-liver-and-gastrointestinal-tract/constipation

8. Courtney E. Ackerman, MA. (2023, September 22). *Mindfulness-Based Stress Reduction: The Ultimate MBSR Guide.* PositivePsychology.com. https://positivepsychology.com/mindfulness-based-stress-reduction-mbsr/

9. Department of Health & Human Services. (1999, May 18). *Crohn's disease and ulcerative colitis.* Better Health Channel. https://www.betterhealth.vic.gov.au/health/conditionsandtreatments/crohns-disease-and-ulcerative-colitis

10. Edermaniger, L. (2022, March 9). *How to improve gut health: 16 simple hacks for your gut in 2022.* Atlas Biomed blog | Take control of your health with no-nonsense news on lifestyle, gut microbes and genetics. https://atlasbiomed.com/blog/16-easy-hacks-to-enhance-your-gut-health-every-day-in-2020/

11. Evenepoel, P., Dejongh, S., Verbeke, K., & Meijers, B. (2020).

The Role of Gut Dysbiosis in the Bone–Vascular Axis in Chronic Kidney Disease. Toxins, 12(5), 285. https://doi.org/10.3390/toxins12050285

12. *Foods linked to better brainpower.* Harvard Health. (2021, March 6). https://www.health.harvard.edu/healthbeat/foods-linked-to-better-brainpower

13. *Gastroesophageal reflux disease (GERD).* Johns Hopkins Medicine. (n.d.). https://www.hopkinsmedicine.org/health/conditions-and-diseases/gastroesophageal-reflux-disease-gerd

14. Gina Simmons Schneider, Ph. D. (2022, August 26). *This is exactly how anxiety can harm your gut microbiome, from a therapist.* mindbodygreen. https://www.mindbodygreen.com/articles/gut-health-mental-health-connection

15. Gis. (2021, June 1). *Your gut microbiota – balanced or not? - Gastrointestinal Society.* Gastrointestinal Society. https://badgut.org/information-centre/a-z-digestive-topics/gut-microbiota-balanced/#:~:text=Research%20shows%20that%20gut%20microorganisms,this%20state%20is%20called%20normobiosis

16. *Go with your gut: Gut health quiz.* Benenden Health. (2023, May 5). https://www.benenden.co.uk/be-healthy/body/go-with-your-gut-quiz/

17. Goodreads. (n.d.). *The mind-gut connection quotes by Emeran Mayer.* Goodreads. https://www.goodreads.com/work/quotes/44319543-the

-mind-gut-connection-how-the-astonishing-dialogue-taking-place-in-ou

18. *Gut Health and nutrient absorption*. Ixcela. (n.d.). https://ixcela.com/resources/gut-health-and-nutrient-absorption.html

19. *Gut health quiz*. The Gut Health Doctor. (2023, August 25). https://www.theguthealthdoctor.com/gut-health-quiz

20. *Gut Stats & Gut Facts: All about gut health*. Pendulum. (n.d.). https://pendulumlife.com/blogs/news/gut-stats-gut-facts-all-about-gut-health

21. Harvard Health. (2021, March 6). *Foods linked to better brainpower*. https://www.health.harvard.edu/healthbeat/foods-linked-to-better-brainpower

22. *Inflammatory bowel disease clinic*. Supported by the University of Alberta. (n.d.). http://www.ibdclinic.ca/what-is-ibd/digestive-system-and-its-function/why-is-digestion-important/

23. Jennings, K.-A. (2023, January 23). *11 best foods to boost your brain and memory*. Healthline. https://www.healthline.com/nutrition/11-brain-foods

24. JHoldsworth. (2020, August 24). *The Gut Quiz*. Guts UK. https://gutscharity.org.uk/2020/02/the-gut-quiz/

25. Kubala, J. (2023, June 16). *The 8 most common food intolerances*. Healthline. https://www.healthline.com/nutrition/common-food-intolerances

26. *Lactose intolerance*. Lactose Intolerance | Boston Children's Hospital. (n.d.). https://www.childrenshospital.org/conditions/lactose-intolerance

27. Lauren Armstrong, R. (2020, July 14). *From food to poo: How long does digestion take?*. Greatist. https://greatist.com/health/how-long-does-it-take-to-digest-food

28. Makinde, S. (2023, April 17). *What are the signs of a healthy digestive system?*. Perfect Balance Clinic. https://www.perfectbalanceclinic.com/what-are-the-signs-of-a-healthy-digestive-system/

29. Mayo Foundation for Medical Education and Research. (2021, February 23). *Hiatal hernia*. Mayo Clinic. https://www.mayoclinic.org/diseases-conditions/hiatal-hernia/symptoms-causes/syc-20373379

30. Mayo Foundation for Medical Education and Research. (2022, April 28). *Relaxation techniques: Try these steps to reduce stress*. Mayo Clinic. https://www.mayoclinic.org/healthy-lifestyle/stress-management/in-depth/relaxation-technique/art-20045368

31. Mayo Foundation for Medical Education and Research. (2023, August 22). *Diarrhea*. Mayo Clinic. https://www.mayoclinic.org/diseases-conditions/diarrhea/symptoms-causes/syc-20352241

32. Mayo Foundation for Medical Education and Research. (2023a, January 4). *Gastroesophageal reflux disease (GERD)*. Mayo Clinic. https://www.mayoclinic.org/diseases-conditi

ons/gerd/symptoms-causes/syc-20361940

33. Mayo Foundation for Medical Education and Research. (2023a, March 2). *Colon polyps*. Mayo Clinic. https://www.mayoclinic.org/diseases-conditions/colon-polyps/symptoms-causes/syc-20352875

34. Mayo Foundation for Medical Education and Research. (2023c, May 12). *Irritable bowel syndrome*. Mayo Clinic. https://www.mayoclinic.org/diseases-conditions/irritable-bowel-syndrome/symptoms-causes/syc-20360016

35. Mayo Foundation for Medical Education and Research. (n.d.). *Lactose intolerance*. Mayo Clinic. https://www.mayoclinic.org/diseases-conditions/lactose-intolerance/symptoms-causes/syc-20374232

36. Mayo Foundation for Medical Education and Research. (n.d.-a). *Gallstones*. Mayo Clinic. https://www.mayoclinic.org/diseases-conditions/gallstones/symptoms-causes/syc-20354214

37. MediLexicon International. (n.d.). *Food intolerance: Causes, types, symptoms, and diagnosis*. Medical News Today. https://www.medicalnewstoday.com/articles/263965#

38. MediLexicon International. (n.d.-a). *Common digestive disorders: Symptoms and treatments*. Medical News Today. https://www.medicalnewstoday.com/articles/list-of-digestive-disorders

39. Millar, A. (2021, November 1). *What's the link between anxiety and Gut Health?* Patient.info

. https://patient.info/news-and-features/whats-the-link-between-anxiety-and-gut-health

40. Northwestern Medicine. (n.d.). *Celiac disease vs. gluten intolerance (infographic)*. https://www.nm.org/healthbeat/healthy-tips/celiac-disease-vs-gluten-intolerance-infographic

41. Novak, S. (2023, July 21). *Revealed: The five foods that are key to maintaining good gut health*. New Scientist. https://www.newscientist.com/article/2383723-revealed-the-five-foods-that-are-key-to-maintaining-good-gut-health/

42. Orenstein, B. W., Iliades, C., Fritz, A. L., Rapaport, L., Welch, A., Scott, J. A., Marks, J. L., Patino, E., & Rauf, D. (n.d.). *9 common digestive conditions from top to bottom*. EverydayHealth.com. https://www.everydayhealth.com/digestive-health/common-digestive-conditions-from-top-bottom/

43. Plevin, D., Galletly, C. The neuropsychiatric effects of vitamin C deficiency: a systematic review. *BMC Psychiatry* **20**, 315 (2020). https://doi.org/10.1186/s12888-020-02730-w

44. Polak K, Bergler-Czop B, Szczepanek M, Wojciechowska K, Frątczak A, Kiss N. Psoriasis and Gut Microbiome-Current State of Art. Int J Mol Sci. 2021 Apr 26;22(9):4529. doi: 10.3390/ijms22094529. PMID: 33926088; PMCID: PMC8123672.

45. professional, C. C. medical. (n.d.). *Digestive system: Function, Organs & Anatomy*. Cleveland Clinic. https://my.cle

velandclinic.org/health/body/7041-digestive-system

46. professional, C. C. medical. (n.d.-b). *Diverticulitis*. Cleveland Clinic. https://my.clevelandclinic.org/health/diseases/10352-diverticulitis

47. professional, C. C. medical. (n.d.-b). *Gastrointestinal diseases: Symptoms, treatment & causes*. Cleveland Clinic. https://my.clevelandclinic.org/health/articles/7040-gastrointestinal-diseases

48. professional, C. C. medical. (n.d.-b). *Gluten intolerance: Symptoms, test, non-celiac gluten sensitivity*. Cleveland Clinic. https://my.clevelandclinic.org/health/diseases/21622-gluten-intolerance

49. professional, C. C. medical. (n.d.-b). *Perianal abscess: Vs. hemorrhoid, causes & treatment, surgery*. Cleveland Clinic. https://my.clevelandclinic.org/health/diseases/23282-perianal-abscess

50. professional, C. C. medical. (n.d.-c). *Gastroparesis*. Cleveland Clinic. https://my.clevelandclinic.org/health/diseases/15522-gastroparesis

51. professional, C. C. medical. (n.d.-c). *Irritable bowel syndrome: IBS, symptoms, causes, treatment*. Cleveland Clinic. https://my.clevelandclinic.org/health/diseases/4342-irritable-bowel-syndrome-ibs

52. professional, C. C. medical. (n.d.-d). *Inflammatory bowel disease: Symptoms, treatment & diagnosis*. Cleveland Clinic. https://my.clevelandclinic.org/health/diseases/155

87-inflammatory-bowel-disease-overview

53. professional, C. C. medical. (n.d.-i). *Stomach cancer: Causes, symptoms, diagnosis & treatment*. Cleveland Clinic. https://my.clevelandclinic.org/health/diseases/15812-stomach-cancer

54. professional, C. C. medical. (n.d.-j). *What to know about the gut-brain connection*. Cleveland Clinic. https://my.clevelandclinic.org/health/body/the-gut-brain-connection

55. Rdn, C. C. (2024, February 26). The secret of serotonin and gut health - My good gut. *My Good Gut*. https://mygoodgut.com/serotonin-and-gut-health/

56. Robertson, R. (2023, April 3). *How does your gut microbiome impact your overall health?*. Healthline. https://www.healthline.com/nutrition/gut-microbiome-and-health

57. Rodrigues, F. G., Ormanji, M. S., Heilberg, I. P., Bakker, S. J. L., & de Borst, M. H. (2021). Interplay between gut microbiota, bone health and vascular calcification in chronic kidney disease. European journal of clinical investigation, 51(9), e13588. https://doi.org/10.1111/eci.13588

58. Sanchez, M. (2023, October 5). *What your poop says about your health*. HealthPartners Blog. https://www.healthpartners.com/blog/healthy-poop-chart/

59. Sarah. (2021, October 11). *8 lifestyle habits destroying your gut health*. Gut Performance. https://gutperformance.com.au/8-lifestyle-habits-destroying-your-gut-health/

60. Segula, D., Mwandiambira, V., Howson, W., & Allain, T. J. (2011). Case report--the 46 year old man with a 5 month history of vomiting. Malawi medical journal : the journal of Medical Association of Malawi, 23(2), 55–57. https://doi.org/10.4314/mmj.v23i2.70752

61. Sikora M, Stec A, Chrabaszcz M, Knot A, Waskiel-Burnat A, Rakowska A, Olszewska M, Rudnicka L. Gut Microbiome in Psoriasis: An Updated Review. Pathogens. 2020 Jun 12;9(6):463. doi: 10.3390/pathogens9060463. PMID: 32545459; PMCID: PMC7350295.

62. Spend, E. (2022, June 28). Why you need prebiotics, probiotics and postbiotics: The trifecta of good gut health. BodyBio. https://bodybio.com/blogs/blog/prebiotics-vs-probiotics-vs-postbiotics

63. *Success stories*. Be Gut Happy. (n.d.). https://www.beguthappy.co.uk/success-stories

64. *Success stories*. Heal Well Nutrition. (2021, June 13). https://www.healwellnutrition.com/success-stories/

65. *Success story leaky gut health check– verisana labs*. Verisana. (2019, November 23). https://www.verisana.com/about-verisana/success-story-leaky-gut/

66. Sussex Publishers. (n.d.). *The three channels of gut-brain communication*. Psychology Today. https://www.psychologytoday.com/us/blog/mood-by-microbe/202307/the-three-channels-of-gut-brain-communication

67. Sydney Sprouse. (2022, July 20). *Your guide to how nutrients are absorbed by the body*. Ask The Scientists. https://askthescientists.com/nutrient-absorption/

68. *Taking good care of yourself*. Mental Health America. (n.d.). https://mhanational.org/taking-good-care-yourself

69. *The brain-gut connection*. Johns Hopkins Medicine. (2021, November 1). https://www.hopkinsmedicine.org/health/wellness-and-prevention/the-brain-gut-connection

70. *The Gut Brain Connection: How Gut Health Affects Mental Health - PsyCom*. The Gut Brain Connection: How Gut Health Affects Mental Health. (n.d.). https://www.psycom.net/the-gut-brain-connection

71. *The gut-brain axis: How your gut affects your mental health*. CNET. (n.d.). https://www.cnet.com/health/nutrition/the-gut-brain-axis-how-your-gut-affects-your-mental-health/

72. *The relationship between Gut Health and Anxiety*. KnowYourDNA. (2023, January 13). https://knowyourdna.com/gut-health-and-anxiety/

73. U.S. Department of Health and Human Services. (2018, October 16). *Gut communicates directly with brain*. National Institutes of Health. https://www.nih.gov/news-events/nih-research-matters/gut-communicates-directly-brain

74. U.S. Department of Health and Human Services. (2022, July 15). *Gut troubles*. National Institutes of Health. https://newsinhealth.nih.gov/2020/02/gut-troubles

75. U.S. Department of Health and Human Services. (2022b, August 8). *Emotional wellness toolkit*. National Institutes of Health. https://www.nih.gov/health-information/emotional-wellness-toolkit

76. U.S. Department of Health and Human Services. (n.d.). *Your digestive system & how it works - niddk*. National Institute of Diabetes and Digestive and Kidney Diseases. https://www.niddk.nih.gov/health-information/digestive-diseases/digestive-system-how-it-works

77. U.S. Department of Health and Human Services. (n.d.-a). *Acid reflux (ger & gerd) in adults - niddk*. National Institute of Diabetes and Digestive and Kidney Diseases. https://www.niddk.nih.gov/health-information/digestive-diseases/acid-reflux-ger-gerd-adults

78. U.S. Department of Health and Human Services. (n.d.-a). *Your digestive system & how it works - niddk*. National Institute of Diabetes and Digestive and Kidney Diseases. https://www.niddk.nih.gov/health-information/digestive-diseases/digestive-system-how-it-works

79. U.S. Department of Health and Human Services. (n.d.-b). *Diverticular disease - NIDDK*. National Institute of Diabetes and Digestive and Kidney Diseases. https://www.niddk.nih.gov/health-information/digestive-diseases/diverticulosis-diverticulitis#:~:text=Diverticulosis%20is%20a%20condition%20that,call%20this%20condition%20diverticular%20disease

80. U.S. Department of Health and Human Services. (n.d.-b).

Gastroparesis - niddk. National Institute of Diabetes and Digestive and Kidney Diseases. https://www.niddk.nih.gov/health-information/digestive-diseases/gastroparesis

81. U.S. Department of Health and Human Services. (n.d.-b). *Symptoms & causes of celiac disease - NIDDK*. National Institute of Diabetes and Digestive and Kidney Diseases. https://www.niddk.nih.gov/health-information/digestive-diseases/celiac-disease/symptoms-causes

82. *Ulcerative colitis case study*. Immunopaedia. (2022, December 5). https://www.immunopaedia.org.za/clinical-cases/gastrointestinal-disorders/a-case-of-persistent-bloody-diarrhoea/

83. Wang, R., Li, Z., Liu, S., & Zhang, D. (2023). Global, regional, and national burden of 10 digestive diseases in 204 countries and territories from 1990 to 2019. *Frontiers in Public Health, 11*. https://doi.org/10.3389/fpubh.2023.1061453

84. Watson, S. (2020, April 1). *How long does it take to digest food?*. Healthline. https://www.healthline.com/health/how-long-does-it-take-to-digest-food

85. WebMD. (n.d.). *Anal abscess: Symptoms, causes, and treatments*. WebMD. https://www.webmd.com/a-to-z-guides/anal-abscess

86. Wojtowecz, A. (2021, October 6). *What is the gut-brain axis? how gut health affects mental health*. Well.Org. https://well.org/healthy-body/what-is-gut-brain-axis/

87. *Your serotonin gut health connection.* Dr. Will Cole. (2022, August 30). https://drwillcole.com/gut-health/your-serotonin-gut-health-connection

88. Zhang, Y. J., Li, S., Gan, R. Y., Zhou, T., Xu, D. P., & Li, H. B. (2015). Impacts of gut bacteria on human health and diseases. International journal of molecular sciences, 16(4), 7493–7519. https://doi.org/10.3390/ijms16047493

Understanding Hormones for Women

Simple Steps to Avoid Complications, Reduce Medical Expenses, Decrease Stress and Live a Healthy & Proactive Life

Written By Dr. Ashley Sullivan PharmD

Contents

Introduction #

1. The Hormonal Symphony #
2. The Monthly Melody #
3. Decoding the Body's Distress Signals #
4. Unmasking Hormone Tests #
5. Nourishing Your Hormones #

Share Your Light #

6. Herbs at Your Service #
7. Balancing Act #
8. The Fertility Mystery #
9. Conquering Hormonal Challenges #
10. Your Map to Harmonious Hormones #

Conclusion #

Small Act, Big Impact #

References

Introduction

The Importance of a Holistic Approach to Hormonal Imbalance

In what should be the prime of life, women often find themselves grappling with an unexpected adversary—hormonal imbalances.

Picture this: a woman is standing before the mirror, hesitating, fearing what she may see reflected back. Her confidence is already shattered by painful cyst-like acne that no amount of makeup can conceal. And now there are relentless battles with unwanted body hair, sprouting in places it has no business being.

Thick, dark stubble on her chin, legs, and stomach leads to a relentless routine of shaving and hair removal creams. But the physical manifestations are just the tip of the iceberg.

Weight gain starts to seem inevitable, as if merely breathing in air or catching a whiff of cooked food will pile on the pounds. And as if that isn't enough, her periods become increasingly agonizing and frequent, leaving her feeling drained and hopeless.

Faced with this uphill battle, she tries everything within her power to regain control of her body. From birth control to painkillers, she seeks solace in temporary fixes that only offer fleeting relief. And yet, the root cause remains elusive.

Going through this alone as a woman is difficult and depressing, especially if family and friends cannot relate to the symptoms. But armed with determination, she decides to embark on a quest for holistic healing, determined to reclaim her well-being and defy the odds that are seemingly stacked against her. And with her newfound knowledge, she discovers the importance of advocating for herself in the face of dismissive medical professionals.

There are currently millions of women going through similar issues, deeply insecure, with no one to talk to. About 80 percent of women around the world suffer from hormonal imbalances. Some even live with it without realizing it, unaware of conditions like PCOS that they may be currently experiencing as a result of hormone irregularities.

As a pharmacist and integrative health coach with a deep understanding of pharmaceuticals underpinning my holistic approach to health and wellness, I am passionate about helping women just like you achieve hormonal balance naturally. Based on my personal experiences and expertise, I can provide you with the knowledge and tools to regain control over your hormonal health, which will have a powerful impact on your quality of life.

I have attended countless seminars and workshops, read books specializing in this area, and interacted with different women facing the same issues I have faced with hormones; and I have discovered and learned a lot.

Conventional medicine can be one-dimensional, often resulting in treatment by medication. This method treats hormonal imbalance as something that needs to be fixed to relieve symptoms, with little to no attention given to the underlying cause. Every woman is unique, and so is her hormonal balance. Understanding and effectively treating hormonal imbalance requires a whole-body approach, which involves taking an all-encompassing 360-degree view of your health and looking at your whole person—not just separate organs or body systems.

Often, women feel helpless trying to explain their symptoms to doctors, who only end up offering a "one size fits all" approach like hormone replacement therapy (HRT) or antidepressants. This is not the best option to resolve hormonal imbalance symptoms.

I know from my experience that these symptoms can also be overwhelming, which again shows the importance of having a doctor who takes time to understand before proposing solutions. The reality is that not all of us have a doctor we feel comfortable confiding in and guiding us. One that doesn't take the approach of brushing all complaints under the rug. This is why the holistic approach of listening to your concerns and taking your whole body into consideration is so much better.

The Importance of Understanding Our Hormones

Are you aware that our bodies possess the innate ability to maintain a healthy balance of hormones throughout our lives? It's hard to believe, isn't it? All the body needs is a nudge in the right direction so it can carry out this task on an ongoing basis.

As the body's messenger, your hormones are a part of the endocrine system, a vast network of communication that regulates all the biological processes in the body, including metabolism and growth. It also affects your mental, emotional, and physical health. Endocrine glands, which are special groups of cells, secrete hormones. Hormones have great power; even small amounts can alter cells or possibly your entire body in a significant way. So, when there is an imbalance, whether it is too high or too low, it can result in a series of problems and serious changes like weight gain, irritability, and other health issues.

This book not only enlightens women on their hormones but also serves as a resource for women battling hormonal imbalances, emphasizing the impact of nutrition on emotional and hormonal health. You'll also learn that no matter your age or marital status, whether you work full-time or are a stay-at-home mom, embracing a holistic approach to balancing your hormones will make an incredible difference, affecting a positive change in your overall health and well-being. The investment you have made in yourself by reading this book will continue to grow as you apply the knowledge gained here to empower yourself and take control of your hormonal health—the holistic and least invasive way.

In the chapters that follow, I will provide you with practical and credible advice on lifestyle changes, dietary modifications, and natural remedies. I will introduce you to ten steps that are necessary for understanding your hormonal health as a woman. These steps focus on comprehensive coverage of fundamental principles, various hormonal issues and their impact on women's health, personal stories from women I have had the opportunity to interact with on this subject, meal plans, and personalized solutions to achieve optimal well-being in your life and the lives of other women around you.

If you want to make a positive change in your hormonal health using a holistic approach, you are going to need to be committed enough to work at it. This book will serve as a guide toward helping you achieve your goal. I will provide you with all the necessary information, but then it's up to you to put in effort and discipline.

I did not come to this knowledge overnight. Every piece of information in this book is supported by scientific research and my years of professional experience. I have broken everything down into small bites of information and tailored it specifically to the unique hormonal health challenges that women face. Remember, this is an investment in you. I wish you the best as you use this book as your guide and companion on your path to hormonal health.

And to every woman out there struggling with hormonal imbalance, I want you to know—you are not alone.

Chapter One

The Hormonal Symphony

An Overview of Hormones and Their Function

Hormonal imbalance is normal; it is one of the ups and downs of being a woman.

This is a common myth passed through society with no credibility. I grew up hearing it from my teachers and friends and was forced to accept that as my stark reality. Well, I am here to debunk that rumor. While hormonal imbalance is common, it's not normal. If you've been dealing with your reproductive health, issues with fertility, or overly painful menstruation, the subject of hormones and their function will have come up a lot. But, in order to ensure you fully understand what hormones are and how they function in your body, we will spend some time focusing on this before we dive into hormonal balances and their root causes.

The Role of Hormones in the Body

The human body is made up of an intricate network of structures that interact with the brain. One of the most important structures of the body is the hormone system. Hormones act like little chemical messengers, helping to run bodily functions, from simple needs like hunger and metabolizing food to complex systems like reproduction, mood, and emotions. They are secreted directly into the blood, which then transports them directly to various organs and tissues in the body where they carry out their duties and modify other bodily functions.

These hormones are secreted from the endocrine "ductless" glands. These glands do not release their secretions into ducts, or tubes, but instead release the hormones directly into the bloodstream. This is beneficial because it allows the hormones to be available in the bloodstream for efficient distribution throughout the body. This ductless system enables hormones to quickly reach their target tissues and organs, facilitating precise regulation and coordination of various physiological processes.

Major organs and cells in the body secrete hormones for various functions, and these hormones normally become by-products after the body has metabolized them. It's an incredibly complex system, which is why your overall health and well-being depend on a balanced and healthy hormonal system.

Different hormones perform specific roles inside your body. According to endocrinologists, hormones regulate metabolism, respiration, growth, reproduction, sensory perception, and movement. They also help in the maintenance of body temperature, thirst, cognitive function, and mood (Dr. Robert Lustig Website 2024).

Hormones can also influence the immune system and even behaviors, as underscored in research by neuropsychologist Dr. Robert Sapolsky. This interaction is bidirectional: Hormones can affect behavior, and in turn, behavior can influence hormone concentrations.

According to Dr. Hermann, a psychiatrist at Weill Cornell Medicine, hormones have a vast impact on mood and anxiety. She explains how estrogen can act as an antidepressant chemical in the brain, how having too high or too low thyroid levels can cause depression and anxiety, and also how the stress hormone cortisol affects mood (*Hormones' Role on Our Health, and Wellness | Patient Care*, 2019).

Hormones also play a significant role in our emotional well-being, anxiety levels, and overall mental health, as highlighted in numerous studies in the "Journal of Psychiatry and Neuroscience." For example, during the menstrual cycle, fluctuations in estrogen and progesterone levels can lead to PMS symptoms. In some women, these hormonal shifts tend to contribute to mood swings, increased irritability, and emotional sensitivity.

Pregnancy also comes with a surge of hormones, including human chorionic gonadotropin (HCG) and progesterone, which can affect mood. Some pregnant women relate being depressed or facing mood swings during their pregnancy, while others experience euphoria.

As for menopause, there is a steep decline in the levels of estrogen and progesterone produced by the body; this can result in frequent anxiety, hot flashes, mood swings, and bouts of depression. It's important to understand that hormonal changes can significantly impact our mental and emotional state. Being aware of these potential effects can help us better manage our well-being during different life stages and seek support when needed.

Another example is the "feel-good" hormone, serotonin, which helps regulate mood and social behavior, appetite and digestion, sleep, memory, sexual desire, and function.

When these hormones are in proper balance, they help the body thrive, but small problems with them can cause severe symptoms. "The brain can adjust and be okay with high or low hormones; where it gets into trouble is when the hormones are changing all the time. Some women are more sensitive than others," states Dr. Hermann.

With hormones, it takes only a small amount to cause big changes in your body. This minor change in hormone levels can cause a significant change to the body, which can sometimes lead to medical conditions that then need treatment.

Scientists have identified over fifty hormones present in the human body. However, according to their chemical makeup, these hormones can be broadly classified into three categories:

Lipid-derived hormones (or lipid-soluble hormones): These hormones are transported through the body in the bloodstream by transport proteins. Most lipid hormones are derived from cholesterol and are structurally similar to it. The primary class of lipid hormones is steroid hormones. Examples of steroid hormones include estradiol, which is a type of female sex hormone (estrogen), and hormones released by the adrenal glands, namely cortisol and aldosterone, which are in charge of regulating bodily functions such as metabolism and the body's response to stress.

Peptide hormones: Peptide hormones, also known as protein hormones, have been implicated in controlling appetites, gastrointestinal and cardiovascular systems, energy expenditure, and reproduction. Some examples of these types of hormones include insulin, follicle-stimulating hormone (FSH), human growth hormone (HGH), pituitary hormones, and thyroid hormones (T3 and T4).

Amino acid-derived hormones: Many of these hormones are neurotransmitters that send messages between nerve cells in the nervous system. If a hormone is amino acid-derived, its chemical name will end in "-ine." Examples include epinephrine and norepinephrine.

The Endocrine System: the Conductor of the Hormonal Orchestra

The endocrine system is the body's network of glands that produce, store, and secrete hormones into the bloodstream. As I mentioned earlier, these hormones control many vital functions in the body. There are many different glands within the endocrine system, and each gland produces specific hormones that play a unique and vital role in regulating various bodily functions.

Glands and Hormones in the Body

The following organs and glands make up your endocrine system, together with some of the different hormones they produce and secrete in the body:

- Pituitary gland
- Thyroid gland
- Parathyroid glands
- Adrenal gland
- Pineal gland
- Hypothalamus
- Pancreas
- Ovaries

Pituitary gland: This gland is located at the base of the brain, behind the bridge of your nose, and directly below your hypothalamus. It is often referred to as the system's "master control gland." The pituitary gland consists of two main sections: the anterior and posterior lobes. Together, these two lobes produce eight hormones. The anterior pituitary (front lobe) is responsible for creating and releasing six main hormones. Namely, adrenocorticotropic hormone (ACTH), follicle-stimulating hormone (FSH), luteinizing hormone (LSH), growth hormone (GH), prolactin, and thyroid-stimulating hormone (TSH). The posterior pituitary (back lobe) secretes two hormones—antidiuretic hormone (ADH) and oxytocin.

- **Growth hormone**: The pituitary gland secretes small amounts of the human chorionic gonadotropin (HCG) hormone. The growth hormone tends to stimulate the release of eggs during ovulation. It's important to note that the level of this growth hormone usually surges during pregnancy and is responsible for bone and muscle growth, as well as cell reproduction.

- **Thyroid-stimulating hormone:** This hormone regulates the thyroid gland. It stimulates the thyroid to produce thyroid hormones that regulate metabolism, heart rate, body temperature, energy levels, and the nervous system. By doing this, it helps to ensure optimal levels of thyroid hormone in your body. If it's too high, it can cause hyperthyroidism; whereas too little thyroid hormone can cause hypothyroidism.

- **Adrenocorticotropic hormone (ACTH):** This hormone regulates the adrenal glands. The adrenal glands are known for producing hormones involved in stress response, metabolism, and blood pressure regulation. The adrenocorticotropic hormone governs the production of *cortisol*, also known as the "stress hormone." Overproduction of this stress hormone can be harmful to the body, resulting in a condition known as Cushing's syndrome. The abuse of steroid medications is a common cause of this disorder.

- **Follicle-stimulating hormone (FSH):** As a woman, this hormone is essential for your reproductive organs. It plays a significant role in sexual development and reproduction by affecting the function of your ovaries and developing eggs. It works alongside the luteinizing hormone and plays different roles at different stages of your life. For example, the follicle-stimulating hormone helps regulate the menstrual cycle by stimulating follicles on the ovary to grow and prepare for ovulation. Also, in the second and third trimesters of pregnancy, FSH levels peak, playing a vital role in fetal development.

☐ **Luteinizing hormone (LH):** Another hormone that is very important in the reproductive system, allowing it to function correctly, is luteinizing hormone. It stimulates processes in your body that are important for sexual health, development, and reproduction. Luteinizing hormone is involved in the process of ovulation in women and helps with hormone production needed to support pregnancy. LH levels also act as a signal for diagnosing reproductive health issues like fertility, irregular periods, and how close you are to perimenopause and menopause. As you age and go through menopause, your LH levels will increase as your levels of estrogen and progesterone decrease.

☐ **Prolactin:** Prolactin is involved in the development of the mammary glands, lactation, and the production of milk in the body. This hormone is normally at its peak in pregnant women and breastfeeding women.

☐ **Vasopressin (an antidiuretic hormone):** This hormone regulates water balance in the body by regulating water excretion from the kidney.

☐ **Oxytocin:** Sometimes called the "cuddle hormone," it's responsible for bonding, reproduction, and lactation.

Thyroid gland: The thyroid gland is a small, butterfly-shaped gland located in the neck. Its primary job involves regulating body temperature, speed of metabolism, and heart rate. It produces four hormones. Namely:

- Thyroxine (T3)

- Triiodothyronine (T4)

- Calcitonin

- Reverse triiodothyronine (RT3)

Parathyroid glands: This gland is mostly located behind your thyroid gland in your neck, but can sometimes be found along your esophagus or in your chest. The parathyroid gland secretes the *parathyroid hormone*, which is responsible for ensuring calcium balance in your blood and bones.

Adrenal glands: These glands are located on the kidneys and produce hormones that play vital roles in how the body responds to stress, as well as in how it regulates metabolism and blood pressure. They produce the following hormones:

- DHEA and androgens

- Aldosterone

- Adrenaline (epinephrine) and

- Noradrenaline (norepinephrine)

One of the most important hormones the adrenal glands produce is the *androgen* hormone. Androgens are male sex hormones, but they can also be present in small amounts in women.

The most important androgen is testosterone, which is in charge of developing male characteristics such as muscle and bone mass. It also regulates the development of the male reproductive system. Men and women make testosterone in different organs. In men, it is produced in the testicles, while in women, it is produced in the adrenal glands.

Female bodies readily convert this testosterone hormone into the female sex hormone, estrogen.

Generally, women's bodies make about one-tenth to one-twentieth of the amount of testosterone made by men's bodies. However, during puberty, when there is a surge of testosterone in women, the body can find it difficult to keep converting it to estrogen, resulting in some women developing more male secondary sex characteristics, such as facial hair.

Pineal gland: The pineal gland is located in your brain. Its primary function involves the secretion of the hormone *melatonin*, which helps control your sleep-wake cycle.

Hypothalamus: The hypothalamus is the primary regulator of the pituitary gland. It senses the level of hormones in the body, signaling the pituitary gland to release several hormones, which in turn control the function of other endocrine glands. Some of the hormones include:

- Corticotrophin-releasing hormone
- Dopamine
- Growth hormone-releasing hormone
- Oxytocin
- Somatostatin
- Thyrotropin-releasing hormone
- Gonadotrophin-releasing hormone

Pancreas: The pancreas is located in the abdomen, and it produces hormones that help regulate blood sugar levels, such as *insulin* and *glucagon*. Insulin regulates blood sugar levels by helping the body store and use glucose (sugar).

Ovaries: These are located in the pelvic area, and they produce two main hormones: ***estrogen*** and ***progesterone***. Estrogen is involved in the development of female sexual characteristics and the regulation of the menstrual cycle. Progesterone is involved in preparing the body for pregnancy by thickening the uterus lining. It also plays a role in milk production.

There are many other hormones produced by other glands in the body. These hormones also play essential roles in regulating growth, metabolism, and bone health.

How Does Each Hormone Work in the Body?

When hormones produced by the endocrine glands are secreted into the bloodstream, they tend to travel through the blood to their target organs or tissues. In the human body, hormones are used for communication by sending signals either between two endocrine glands or between an endocrine gland and an organ or tissue. They will only act on a part of your body if it fits; that is, if the cells in the target tissue or gland have receptors that can receive the message of the hormone.

In summary, a balanced endocrine system ensures optimal health and well-being. However, certain factors, like stress, poor nutrition, and illness, can disrupt this balance. When this balance is disrupted, various health issues can arise, as highlighted by the Mayo Clinic's website (Mayo Clinic 2023).

The Importance of Hormonal Balance

A balanced hormonal system is key to overall health. According to the American Association of Clinical Endocrinologists, hormones are involved in almost every function of the body, making hormonal balance essential for good health. For example, the hormone insulin, known for regulating blood sugar levels, helps prevent conditions like diabetes. Oversecretion of insulin can result in severe hypoglycemia, which can lead to seizures and death, while undersecretion of insulin can lead to diabetes.

When you provide your body with the consistent support that it needs, each hormone has clear instructions and the resources to perform its function of keeping you healthy and strong.

Hormonal imbalance can lead to a wide range of health issues, from weight gain and mood swings to more serious conditions like thyroid disease and diabetes. This is also pointed out by Dr. Sara Gottfried in her book *The Hormone Cure*. She states that hormonal imbalances can lead to symptoms like persistent weight gain, fatigue, low libido, anxiety, irritability, depression, and insomnia (Gottfried 2020).

In particular, Gottfried emphasizes how hormonal imbalances can lead to polycystic ovary syndrome (PCOS), endometriosis, and fertility issues in women. For example, there is a standard level of testosterone in women, ranging from 15 to 70 nanograms per deciliter (ng/dL) (Gottfried 2020). When testosterone levels are imbalanced and lower than normal, they may cause fertility problems, vaginal dryness, irregular menstrual periods, and low sex drive. When they become higher than normal, it can result in infertility, PCOS, severe acne, obesity, a lack of menstruation, and excessive hair growth.

These are not fun symptoms to experience, which is why we are on the path to achieving hormonal balance naturally. There are natural foods and herbs that you can incorporate into your diet to help maintain balance naturally, but we will get to that in the oncoming chapters.

Discovering the Reasons for Hormonal Imbalances

Do you find yourself suddenly gaining or losing weight in the blink of an eye? Do you sometimes feel sleep-deprived or like the sleep you get isn't good? Is horrible acne appearing again that refuses to clear up, or do you suffer with dry skin? It could be your hormones at play.

There are lots of possible causes of hormonal imbalance in the body. It can occur due to stress, a poor diet, a lack of exercise, or certain medical conditions. For instance, chronic stress can lead to adrenal fatigue, a condition where the adrenal glands are unable to produce adequate amounts of stress hormones. This then leads to symptoms like fatigue, sleep disturbances, and lower immunity. Poor diet is another common cause of hormonal imbalance. Consuming too much sugar, for example, can lead to insulin resistance, impacting blood sugar levels.

Restoring hormonal balance often requires addressing the root causes. As Dr. Mark Hyman emphasizes in his book *The Blood Sugar Solution*, dietary changes and stress management techniques can significantly help in managing hormonal imbalances. A balanced diet rich in lean proteins, healthy fats, and low-glycemic carbohydrates can help to regulate blood sugar levels and maintain hormonal balance.

Chapter Two

The Monthly Melody

Decoding Your Menstrual Cycle

"*Your menstrual cycle is more than your bleeding.
It carries your ancient wisdom.
It is how we know ourselves deeply.
It is where so much healing occurs.
It is how we return to our womanhood.*"
– Anonymous

Your menstrual cycle isn't just about fertility; neither is it about you focusing on surviving the day as you bleed or being miserable during the entire phase of your cycle. Rather, it's a time for you to bask in your feminine energy, revel in the freedom of your body's timing, and understand and tune into the natural rhythm of your body. It's a month-long series of hormonal ebb and flow with inevitable hormonal fluctuations that are an integral part of your life.

This natural and physiological process involves a delicate dance of hormones, each playing a crucial role in your cycle. The menstrual cycle is a natural process that prepares your body for a possible pregnancy. It begins when you get your period. Otherwise known as menstruation.

What Is Menstruation?

Menstruation is the monthly shedding of your uterine lining. It's also commonly referred to as "a period," "Aunt Flo," "menses," "menstrual cycle," and so many other names. When you menstruate, your body discards the monthly buildup of lining from your uterus. This has been built up over the month in the body's effort to create a thick and spongy nest for pregnancy.

Menstruation is primarily driven by hormones. If the woman does not get pregnant, her hormone levels—estrogen and progesterone—begin falling, and it sends a signal to the body to begin menstruation. The uterine lining is then shed, flowing out from the uterus through the tiny opening in the cervix and out from the vagina. This discharge is tissue from the walls of your uterus mixed with a small amount of blood.

How Long Is the Menstrual Cycle?

The average length of a menstrual cycle is twenty-eight days. It can range in length from twenty-one days to about thirty-five to thirty-eight days and still be considered normal, but each woman is different. For example, some teenagers may have cycles that last forty-five days.

The Four Phases of Your Menstrual Cycle: Nature's Calendar

The rise and fall of your hormones helps to trigger the different phases of your cycle. Your menstrual cycle impacts your mood, energy level, nutritional needs, and your overall well-being. Knowing the phases of the menstrual cycle can help put you in control of your body.

By unraveling the phases and their hormonal intricacies, you can learn to navigate your unique rhythms, take better control of your health, and empower yourself to know when to speak to a doctor.

The menstrual cycle consists of four distinct phases: menstrual, follicular, ovulatory, and luteal.

- **The menstrual phase:** This phase begins on the first day of your period. When no fertilized egg is implanted in the uterus, it triggers a drop in progesterone and estrogen levels. It's characterized by the shedding of the uterine lining, leading to menstrual bleeding. Your period contains blood, mucus, and some cells from the lining of the uterus. Bleeding lasts between three and seven days.

- **The follicular phase:** This phase begins on the first day of your period and lasts for about twelve to fourteen days, ending in ovulation. During this time, the level of the estrogen hormone increases, which causes the uterine lining to grow back and thicken. The pituitary gland in the brain releases follicular-stimulating hormone (FSH) to stimulate the production of several small sacs called follicles on the surface of the ovary. Each of these sacs contains an immature egg, but usually only one follicle will develop into a fully mature egg (the ovum). The rest of the follicles will absorb back into the body. This normally takes place from days ten to fourteen of your cycle. Also, during this phase, your uterus lining thickens again in preparation for pregnancy.

This phase ends when you ovulate.

- **The ovulation phase:** This phase is your most fertile, and it usually takes place on day fourteen of your cycle, about two weeks before your next period. It's characterized by a surge in the luteinizing hormone (LH), which is released as a result of rising estrogen levels in the body. The luteinizing hormone helps stimulate the ovary, leading to the release of the already-mature egg from the ovary along the fallopian tube into the uterus. The eggs can survive for up to twenty-four hours. They can be fertilized at any time during ovulation, if they come in contact with sperm. Progesterone levels are really low in this phase, with a peak in the estrogen hormone.

- **The luteal phase:** In this phase, cells in the ovary (the *corpus luteum*) experience a peak in the progesterone hormone level together with rising estrogen in small amounts. If an egg is fertilized, it implants itself in the thickening lining of the uterus, and the *corpus luteum* continues to produce progesterone. However, if fertilization does not occur, the *corpus luteum* dies, progesterone levels drop, the uterus lining sheds, and the menstrual phase begins again. During the luteal phase, women are susceptible to experiencing premenstrual syndrome (PMS), poor sleep quality, increased irritability, and bloating.

Hormonal Symphony: How Hormones Dance Through Your Cycle

In the book *The Women's Book* Lyle McDonald and Eric Helms show us how, during a woman's menstrual cycle, a lot of changes in hormone levels can cause large-scale shifts in her physiology. Among others, changes can happen in her metabolic rate, the propensity of her body to store fat, the rate at which she gets hungry, and insulin sensitivity.

Different hormones experience a surge or decline at different stages of the menstrual cycle, beautifully choreographing the monthly routine of your body, but we will mostly focus on three. These are:

- **Estrogen:** This is the female sex hormone, also known as the growth hormone. It promotes the development of female genital organs and features. During your menstrual cycle, it normally peaks during the follicular phase, aiding in the growth of the uterine lining and stimulating the release of the luteinizing hormone. There are three primary estrogens present in the body. Namely, estrone (E1), estradiol (E2 or 17 beta-estradiol), and estriol (E3), with each having slightly different effects at different times in a woman's life.

Take estriol, which becomes abundant and highly relevant during pregnancy, and estrone, which becomes relevant after menopause. Estradiol (E2) is the most common and potent type of estrogen that people make in the body, particularly during the reproductive years.

After ovulation, the estrogen hormone drops precipitously. This is followed by a secondary rise in estrogen levels during the luteal phase, which faces a downward decline at the end of the menstrual cycle.

- **Progesterone:** This is the second primary reproductive hormone in women, released from the *corpus luteum*—cells in the ovary—that develop after the release of the egg at ovulation. It's also known as the pregnancy hormone.

Progesterone remains low during the follicular phase of the menstrual cycle and has little to no effect on the body at that time. And then, after ovulation during the luteal phase, progesterone starts to increase, gradually reaching a peak halfway through the cycle before decreasing again before menstruation. This hormone dominates the luteal phase, playing a vital role in maintaining the uterine lining for the implantation of fertilized eggs.

At its height, directly after ovulation, it also causes an increase in women's body temperature (basal body temperature), which can be used to determine your peak fertility. It also brings about an increase in the rate at which you expend energy, as well as your resting metabolic rate, and in the presence of estrogen, it causes an increase in the rate at which you crave high-calorie foods.

- **Cortisol:** This hormone is commonly referred to as the stress hormone. Cortisol follows a daily rhythm rather than a monthly one. During the luteal phase, its balance with progesterone is crucial for mood and energy levels. Stress can mess with your cycle in so many ways.

Everyone reacts to stress differently, with some people being more sensitive than others. Dr. Barbara Levy, a clinical professor of obstetrics and gynecology at the George Washington University School of Medicine and Health Sciences, explains how stressors can affect your brain chemistry and, in turn, your cycle: "When you're stressed, your body releases the hormone *cortisol,* and high levels of this can stop ovulation in its tracks. Ovulation is key to having a period, and this can affect when and if your period starts."

Your Cycle and Your Symptoms: Making Sense of PMS and Other Cycle-Related Issues

Many symptoms women experience throughout their cycle are due to hormonal fluctuations. Understanding these can help you manage and possibly alleviate these symptoms.

- Premenstrual syndrome (PMS) symptoms, like mood swings, bloating, and acne flare-ups, are often due to a drop in estrogen and progesterone levels just before menstruation.

- Mid-cycle pain, or *Mittelschmerz,* happens around ovulation due to the rupture of the ovarian follicle, and it's a handy (though sometimes painful) signal of ovulation.

- Breast tenderness in the luteal phase is due to high progesterone levels, preparing the body for potential pregnancy.

- Premenstrual dysphoric disorder (PMDD) is a severe form of PMS characterized by more intense mood disturbances and physical symptoms that significantly impact daily life.

You may experience other symptoms like joint aches, coordination issues, headaches, exhaustion, increased irritability, and anger issues. A large percentage of women may suffer from hot flashes when nearing menopause, among many other symptoms. Regular exercise and the consumption of healthy meals can help you deal with these symptoms.

Menstrual Disorders

It's important to note that there is truly no such thing as a normal menstrual cycle. There is a general pattern that occurs, but there are still variations within this pattern between any two women. However, in some cases, it's possible for the cycle to become extremely disrupted.

Some women go through their menstrual cycle with little to no concerns. Their period comes and goes like clockwork, starting and stopping at nearly the same time every month. Other women, though, go through a myriad of physical and emotional symptoms prior to and during menstruation.

According to William H. Parker, MD, a clinical professor at the UC San Diego School of Medicine, menstrual disorders are disruptive physical and emotional symptoms that occur just before or during menstruation, including heavy bleeding, missed periods, and unmanageable mood swings.

These symptoms may prove disruptive in your life, preventing you from carrying out everyday activities with ease. Let's go into some further detail.

- **Amenorrhea**: This refers to the absence of menstruation in your menstrual cycle. It's clinically defined as the lack of menstruation for about ninety days or more, with some women not being able to menstruate for extended lengths of time. There are two types of amenorrhea—primary amenorrhea and secondary amenorrhea.

Primary amenorrhea occurs if a woman does not begin menstruating at the age of fifteen or sixteen, while secondary amenorrhea refers to the lack of a menstrual cycle in a woman who has begun menstruating. We will focus on secondary amenorrhea, since this is more likely to be relevant to most readers of this book.

Common causes of secondary amenorrhea may include stress, poor nutrition, some birth control methods like intrauterine devices (IUDs), extreme weight changes, and extreme exercise routines. Medical conditions like pituitary disorders, hormonal imbalances as a result of PCOS, adrenal disorders or hypothyroidism, hypothalamic amenorrhea (a condition where amenorrhea occurs due to an issue with your hypothalamus), obesity, and chronic illnesses like kidney disease or inflammatory bowel disease may also cause secondary amenorrhea.

If you suffer from amenorrhea, it likely can be treated (cause-dependent) and is not a life-threatening issue. Some of these treatments may include following a healthy diet to ensure healthy weight maintenance, stress management techniques, changing the intensity of exercise levels, hormonal treatment, and, in rare cases, surgery.

- **Dysmenorrhea**: This is a medical term for painful menstrual periods. It's common to experience moderate cramping during a period, but if you experience intense and extremely painful menstrual cramps that interfere with your daily activities, then you may suffer from dysmenorrhea.

There are two types of dysmenorrhea: primary and secondary dysmenorrhea. Primary dysmenorrhea is the more common type. If you suffer from primary dysmenorrhea, you will experience mild to severe menstrual cramps in your lower abdomen. This type of dysmenorrhea is recurring, so the pain comes every time you get your period.

Secondary dysmenorrhea is classed as a medical condition, and it occurs when your reproductive organs are affected. For example, endometriosis is a condition where the tissue meant to line your uterus grows outside of it, which could result in swelling, severe cramping, and scarring.

Other medical conditions that could also cause cramping include adenomyosis (a condition where the tissue lining your uterus grows into the muscles of the uterus, causing severe abdominal pain), having a narrowed cervix as a result of surgery, an irregularly shaped uterus, and other medical conditions. Unfortunately, dysmenorrhea cannot be prevented. However, eating healthy and balanced meals coupled with regular exercise may help dull the intensity of menstrual cramps.

- **Menorrhagia**: Do you find yourself passing large blood clots the size of a quarter during your period? Or going through an insane number of sanitary pads during your cycle because you keep soaking through them by the hour? What about the two-step verification method where you double your sanitary products to avoid staining your shorts because of heavy flow? Well, heavy menstrual bleeding is quite a common concern.

Some women experience heavy bleeding during their periods that lasts for more than a few days. A number of conditions may be the cause of heavy menstrual bleeding. Some of these conditions include hormonal imbalance resulting in the endometrium (uterine lining) becoming too thick, thereby releasing a lot of blood when it sheds; non-cancerous growths in your uterus like adenomyosis and polyps; use of hormone-free intrauterine devices; cancer of the uterus or cervix; and other medical conditions like kidney and thyroid disease.

- **Metrorrhagia**: Some women experience irregular or abnormal bleeding between menstrual periods. Sometimes, it may seem as though it follows a pattern and in other cases, it may be totally unpredictable. Hormone levels play a major role in women experiencing irregular bleeding.

Having abnormal periods is not unusual for women who just started menstruating, but as you age, your cycle should become more predictable as your hormones stabilize. So, if you've been menstruating for some time and you are suddenly experiencing erratic menstrual cycles, then it could be a sign of metrorrhagia, with several potential causes like stress, birth control, fertility treatments, nutritional deficiencies, erratic fluctuations in weight, and other underlying health conditions.

- **Fibroids**: These are benign tumors that can develop in the uterus, affecting women in their reproductive and non-reproductive years. They are usually non-cancerous and they vary in size ranging from microscopic to a few inches across. Not all fibroids cause symptoms, but as they get larger, they are more likely to cause symptoms such as heavy menstrual bleeding, pelvic pain, pressure in the lower abdomen, and even pain during sex.

In a study carried out by an acupuncturist and specialist in IVF, Nick Dalton-Brewer, diet and nutrition have been found to play a vital role in reducing the risk of fibroids in women. Diets high in fish; leafy-green vegetables; lean meat like chicken and turkey; citrus fruits; foods rich in vitamin D like salmon, milk, and cereal; and green tea help prevent and inhibit the growth of fibroids.

A diet low in fruits and vegetables and high in alcohol and red meat increases the risk for fibroids. People with a higher body percentage, usually greater than 30 percent, are also at an increased risk of fibroids. So eating healthy, regularly exercising, and maintaining a healthy weight can help reduce your risk for uterine fibroids.

- **Ovarian cysts** are fluid-filled sacs that can develop on the ovaries, sometimes causing pain or discomfort.

Cycle Tracking: Your Personal Health Detective

Tracking your menstrual cycle can provide valuable insights into your hormonal health, allowing you to detect any imbalances early and take action. Noting the length of your cycle, the heaviness of your

UNDERSTANDING LEAKY GUT & HORMONES... 215

bleeding, and any symptoms you experience throughout can help you understand your unique pattern.

Irregular cycles, heavy or painful periods, or severe PMS symptoms are all signs that your hormones may be out of balance. To make cycle tracking easy and to get visual insights into your cycle trends, the use of cycle tracking apps like Clue and Flo is highly recommended.

Cycle Syncing: Harmonizing Your Life with Your Cycle

By understanding your hormonal fluctuations, you can sync your activities to your cycle, optimizing your energy levels, mood, and overall health.

The follicular phase, with its rising estrogen levels, is often a time for creativity, new projects, and socializing. During this phase, you may feel more energized and outgoing, making it an excellent time to start new ventures or connect with others.

The ovulation phase is a high-energy time, great for hard workouts, important meetings, or making big decisions. With a surge of estrogen, you may feel more confident and focused, making it an ideal time to tackle challenging tasks or engage in physical activities.

The luteal phase, with its high progesterone, is a time for slowing down, self-care, and introspection. During this phase, you may feel more introspective and in need of rest. It's a great time to engage in relaxing activities, practice self-care routines, and reflect on your thoughts and emotions.

Menstruation is a time for rest and reflection, where you can listen to your body's need for a slower pace. During this phase, it's essential to be gentle with yourself, prioritize rest, and engage in activities that nourish your mind and body.

By aligning your activities with your body's natural rhythms, you can optimize your energy levels, enhance your productivity, and promote overall well-being. Remember, every woman's cycle is unique, so it's essential to tune in to your body's signals and adjust your routine accordingly.

CHAPTER THREE

Decoding the Body's Distress Signals

Recognizing Signs of Hormonal Imbalance

"In a survey of 2000 American women, aged 30 to 60, it was found that nearly half (47%) of these women have experienced the symptoms of hormonal imbalance, with many unaware of the potential implications of hormones and a vast majority, about 72 per cent, only later understanding the cause of their symptoms"

– Dr. Anna Cabeca, Triple Board OB-GYN

Maintaining homeostasis within the body requires coordination and communication between the cells and tissues in the body. This is achieved through the release of chemicals called hormones. You are meant to feel amazing in your body and bask in your femininity. One of the keys to unlocking this feeling is to balance your hormones.

When you start to balance your hormones, you start to balance your whole life. The signs of hormonal imbalance are so common that it is often mistaken for being normal. Most women around the world fail to recognize that some of the symptoms they experience could be as a result of more than just periodic stress.

It's important to be able to decode your body's distress signals and identify signs of hormonal imbalance. If you can recognize that your hormones are out of sync, then you can optimize your choices to get them back into a synchronous balance.

Listening to Your Body: The Importance of Body Literacy

How in tune are you with your body? Do you easily register slight changes in your body or are you indifferent about it? How compassionate are you about the natural changes your body undergoes?

It's easy to go through life oblivious to your body's needs and what it's trying to tell you when you are dealing with kids, demanding schedules at work, and other daily responsibilities. This can lead to feelings of indifference and neglect about your body's signs for support or change, even affecting what it deems healthy versus what you feel is normal.

The body is constantly giving feedback. Your menstrual cycle, the rate of metabolism, sleep patterns, and mood are all signs of health and wellness. When something is off, it's usually a sign to be watchful and attentive to your body's needs.

This is where body literacy is key; understanding your body and its signals plays a pivotal role in hormonal health.

What is Body Literacy?

Body literacy helps you learn and interpret your body's signals to identify hormonal imbalances early. It refers to the ability to listen to and connect with your body's natural rhythms and functionality to mindfully discern changes. Body literacy helps you feel more knowledgeable and empowered when it comes to your health as a woman.

In simpler terms, by becoming attuned to the unique patterns and changes of your body, you become an active participant in your journey toward health and wellness. Embracing body literacy empowers you to make certain lifestyle modifications, such as prioritizing exercise, nutrition, and self-care. Recognizing symptoms, understanding hormonal shifts, and identifying irregularities will also become second nature.

Body literacy is a combination of three stages: observation, learning, and understanding.

Observation: You can check in with your body and note when there is a change or when something is off. This stage involves giving your body enough time and attention to notice when something feels different or is changing.

But first, you need to be aware of what is currently normal for you. Pay attention to your hormones, taking into consideration the regularity of ovulation and your menstrual cycle, sleep patterns, mood, weight stability or fluctuations, and your regular bowel movements.

Note that whatever you observe in your body may not be necessarily healthy, but this is an essential step in listening to your body.

Learning: To do this, you have to take the observations you made from your body and analyze them so you can draw patterns from them. This helps you respond quickly to changes you notice. Now that you've made certain observations in your body of what you deem currently normal for you, the looming question becomes—are they healthy?

For example, having an irregular menstrual cycle may mean nothing to you. You may even welcome the breaks since periods are no fun. However, having irregular periods over time can signal underlying health issues like polycystic ovary syndrome (PCOS).

Frequent awakenings while sleeping, poor sleep quality, or finding it extremely difficult to fall asleep may be something you have lived with for years, thinking it's normal. But does that make it okay or healthy? Absolutely not!

Understanding: The last step involved in becoming attuned to your body involves your understanding, or being in sync with your body. This makes it easy to receive signals your body sends to you.

Understanding your body allows you to utilize the knowledge to make healthy and informed decisions. It also allows you to take responsibility, leading to an efficient and effective management of your health.

Combining these three phases will help you become more attuned to the needs and changes of your body.

How Do You Become More Body Literate?

You now know to listen more to your body so you can effectively read the changes or signals it sends to you. You also know the steps to take to listen to your body. However, the problem here is you may not know what to listen for or how to react to the messages you receive. In this section, I will help walk you through simple ways you can start to improve your body literacy.

- **Determine the cause and effect:** You can feel more in sync with your body by learning what triggers certain reactions in your body or mind. It could be a change in your diet, an increase in stress levels, or a change in your exercise or sleep routine. For example, if you constantly deal with irregular weight fluctuations, make a note of possible changes. Variance in diet, changes to your schedule, and any areas of stress can all be factors in weight gain or loss.

Doing this will help you to identify and modify potential causes. If you still can't pinpoint the cause, it's advisable to see a physician, as unexplained weight fluctuations may be a sign of underlying medical conditions like polycystic ovary syndrome (PCOS), hypothyroidism, or kidney disease.

- **Symptom and cycle tracking:** Symptom tracking can be done regularly to analyze changes in the body. Apps like Hormone Horoscope can be useful for tracking your symptoms. Cycle tracking is also recommended to help in better understanding your menstrual cycle.

Living in sync with your menstrual cycle empowers you with knowledge about how hormones impact your mood, health, and behavior. It can help you understand why your energy is low on certain cycle days when high progesterone may trigger tiredness. It can aid in planning a pregnancy or in managing PMS symptoms.

Another positive is that you learn to fully harness your hormonal benefits. It helps you to discover the days of your cycle best for scheduling certain activities like first dates, auditions, and interviews, when you're oozing confidence and energy as a result of your hormones in action.

- **Breathwork:** Listening to your breath and learning how to manipulate it can help you manage stress. Stress reduction is one of the immediate benefits of conscious breathing, but it's been found that taking slow, deep breaths offers numerous benefits. These include body relaxation, enhanced digestion, lower blood pressure, better mood, increased quality of sleep, better metabolism, digestion, concentration, and focus.

Pay close attention to your breathing patterns during the day. Do they change depending on the intensity of your activities, your workload, or whomever you interact with? You may gradually learn what puts you in a positive or negative mental space by tuning in.

- **Exercise:** Responding to what your body needs in terms of exercise instead of what you want is quite important. Exercise is closely linked to stress response, so when you overwork your body it triggers the production of excess stress hormone, cortisol.

So, most times, an intense workout may not be what your body needs. For example, yoga classes, a walk, or even sleeping can prove beneficial when you are exhausted.

Focusing on your body and actively listening to its needs may prove challenging at first. Start small and gradually take your time to learn it. Your body speaks its language, and with time and constant practice, you will drastically improve in your body literacy.

It is important, however, to communicate any worrying symptoms—like sleep problems, irregular and painful periods, or unexplained weight gain or loss—effectively to healthcare professionals to ensure you receive appropriate care.

Tell-Tale Signs: Common Symptoms of Hormonal Imbalance

Symptoms of hormonal imbalance can vary widely but there are some common signs:

- **Unexplained weight loss:** Not all weight loss should be a cause for concern. Weight loss can happen after a stressful event or a life-changing, traumatic experience. However, losing weight without even trying may be an indicator of underlying medical conditions. They include:

- **Hyperthyroidism:** The thyroid gland produces the thyroid hormone. It controls many functions in the body, including metabolism. When the thyroid gland makes too much of this hormone, your rate of metabolism will increase. So, even if you have an enormous appetite, you will still quickly burn through calories.

- **Type 1 diabetes:** This is a chronic condition that involves the production of little to no insulin by the pancreas. Insulin is a hormone that the body uses to allow sugar (glucose) to enter cells to produce energy, and without it, your body can't use the glucose for energy. This causes your body to burn fat and muscle for energy, resulting in you losing weight.

- **Depression:** This is a common mood disorder that affects a lot of people, with more women affected than men. This mood disorder affects parts of the brain that control appetite, leading to loss of appetite and weight loss. However, the symptoms may differ from person to person. In some cases, depression can lead to an increase in appetite and weight.

Several other medical conditions can also cause unexplained weight loss, such as inflammatory bowel disease, tuberculosis, cancer, congestive heart failure, and muscle loss.

- **Unexplained weight gain:** Persistent weight gain or trouble losing weight is quite a common and frustrating symptom of hormone imbalance. Many women struggle with rapid weight gain despite working out frequently and dieting. A diverse range of factors related to aging or dietary and lifestyle modifications may lead to weight gain.

For example, when you feel irritated, your estrogen levels drop causing you to want to eat more, resulting in weight gain. However, rapid and unexplained weight gain can indicate issues with insulin, fluctuating levels of the stress hormone cortisol, and the oversecretion or under secretion of thyroid hormones.

Thyroid hormones are particularly known for the active role they play in metabolism in the body. A decrease in the level of secretion of this hormone (hypothyroidism) can cause weight gain.

Rapid weight gain may also be a sign of kidney problems.

- **Chronic fatigue and lack of energy:** Finding it difficult getting up in the morning? Do you constantly feel exhausted and low on energy all the time despite having a good night's sleep? Do you always require caffeine in your system to have a productive day or simply to get through the day? An imbalance in hormones could be the cause.

If the thyroid gland in your neck secretes too little thyroid hormone (hypothyroidism), it results in low energy. Chronic fatigue might also be a sign of adrenal dysfunction. Some studies suggest that long-term stressful situations can overwork the adrenals. In stressful situations, the adrenals can produce excess cortisol to such a degree that the adrenal glands become unable to secrete enough cortisol hormone for optimal body function, resulting in adrenal fatigue.

- **Mood swings and emotional instability:** Mood swings can be linked to imbalances in the female sex hormones estrogen and progesterone. These hormones fluctuate during a woman's cycle. Low estrogen can cause mood changes. A drop in estrogen levels can cause postpartum depression and also depression during perimenopause, which is the time right before menopause begins.

If you suffer from hormonal imbalance, the emotions that you will often feel are those of irritability and sadness. These fluctuations in estrogen levels negatively affect the secretion of happy hormones like serotonin and dopamine. As a result, you are prevented from feeling happy.

- **Chronic acne:** Skin issues like acne breakouts before or during your period are quite common and normal. But if you have chronic acne that refuses to clear up, it could be a symptom of hormonal imbalance. Oversecretion of the androgen hormones—which are considered male hormones but are present in both men and women—causes the skin's oil glands to produce excess oil. This results in clogged pores, which are precursors to acne flare-ups.

- **Dry skin:** During menopause and perimenopause, the level of reproductive hormones that stimulate oil glands reduces. Estrogen is a major player in skin health. It helps stimulate the right amount of oil production needed to keep the skin supple, smooth, and soft.

As we age, the levels of this hormone tend to decline, along with sebum oil production, causing the skin to become dry, rough, and itchy. Glowing skin is a prominent indicator of good health. If you struggle with skin issues like dry skin, it's usually a sign of changes occurring inside your body, and hormonal imbalance could be the reason.

Thyroid hormones also stimulate the production of sebum from oil glands. An imbalance in the secretion of these thyroid hormones—hypothyroidism and hyperthyroidism—usually results in noticeable symptoms like dry skin.

- **Difficulty sleeping:** Sleep is an integral part of a healthy life. It helps the body repair itself and strengthen its immune system. Lack of sleep may interfere with various metabolic processes. Sleep problems are much more likely to be reported by women than men, as they tend to suffer from insomnia more than men.

The hormone estrogen is directly linked to sleep. A decrease in estrogen levels due to physical stress, like over-exercising or dramatic weight loss, may lead to anxiety and sleep disturbance. If you are not getting enough sleep, or find it difficult to sleep, it could be your hormones at play.

Progesterone, a hormone released by the ovaries, also helps you sleep. When the levels of this hormone fall, it can be a cause of sleeplessness, and you may experience difficulty falling asleep. Low levels of estrogen can trigger hot flashes and night sweats, which can make it tough to get the sleep and rest you need.

- **Hair loss:** Lustrous thick hair is a sign of great health. When there is a decrease in the levels of estrogen and progesterone, it prompts an increase in androgen hormones, such as testosterone. As a result, hair follicles shrink, with the hair gradually becoming thinner and less lustrous, leading to complete hair loss. This is particularly noticeable during pregnancy, menopause, or after starting birth control pills.

- **Irregular menstrual cycles:** For some women, their monthly period comes and goes like clockwork, ranging from twenty-one to thirty-five days. Due to certain factors like stress or birth control, a delayed or missed period may occasionally happen. However, if it happens frequently with gaps of several months between each cycle, it could be a sign of hormonal imbalance.

The Bigger Picture: Understanding the Impact of Hormonal Imbalances on Mental Health

"Hormones have a direct connection to how we feel mentally and physically," says Dr. Vasan, MD, psychiatrist and chief medical officer at Real. Almost all your hormones affect your mental health in one way or the other. Hormonal imbalances do not just cause physical symptoms, they significantly impact mental health too (The Link 2024).

The brain and the endocrine system, which produces hormones, are interconnected. Hormones produced by the endocrine glands can directly impact the function of the brain and nervous system.

Serotonin, also known as the happy hormone, is a naturally occurring neurotransmitter that helps regulate your mood and behavior. Imbalances in the secretion of serotonin in your body play a role in certain psychiatric conditions, including anxiety disorders, post-traumatic stress hormone, depressive disorders, and obsessive-compulsive disorder.

Cortisol, commonly referred to as the stress hormone, is a steroid hormone that is involved in the body's response to stress. It can easily get activated, especially when faced with stressful and traumatic situations. High levels of cortisol can exacerbate mental health issues.

Thyroid hormones, secreted from the butterfly-shaped gland in the neck, are known for the major role they play in metabolism. Too little thyroid hormone (hypothyroidism) is linked to low mood or symptoms of depression, while too much thyroid hormone (hyperthyroidism) can cause increased irritability and anxiety.

Imbalances in estrogen and progesterone levels can contribute to mood and irritability issues around your menstrual cycle, postpartum depression following childbirth, and fluctuations in mood during menopause.

Your mental health impacts your behavior, feelings, and thoughts in everyday life. It's also a great barometer for your overall health and well-being. Having good mental health helps you to handle stress and make decisions. You are likely to feel happy, more connected with people, and experience a feeling of satisfaction with life.

Poor mental health can also impact your everyday life, constantly leaving you feeling anxious or worried. It can cause feelings of sadness or depression with occasional emotional outbursts. Most mental health issues—like brain fog, anxiety, or depression—are the result of hormonal imbalance, which is why prioritizing mental health is an essential part of managing hormonal imbalance.

How Can I Regulate My Mental Health and Hormonal Balance?

Making modifications to your lifestyle can go a long way in improving hormonal issues and regulating your mental health.

- **Regular exercise:** When you are stressed, your body releases the stress hormone, cortisol, which can disrupt the action of other hormones present in the body. Regular exercise releases the hormone endorphins that make you feel good. It causes positive changes in your mood, helps relieve feelings of anxiety, and alleviates symptoms of depression.

- **Good sleep:** Poor sleep impacts mental health, making it difficult to cope with stress and decreasing positive emotions. Many of us tend to feel better after a good night's sleep and grumpy after being sleep-deprived. This shows the important role sleep plays in a number of brain and body functions.

- **Dietary modifications:** Eating whole, unprocessed foods and eliminating processed foods is highly recommended for hormonal imbalance. Incorporating a plant-based diet that includes fruits, vegetables, and whole grains into your daily routine will also help provide your body with essential nutrients.

- **Talk therapy:** Ever felt relieved after talking with a loved one? Research shows that engaging in a deep talk with friends, family, or a therapist can help improve your emotional and mental health. Talk therapy is an effective way to reduce anxiety and depression.

- **Meditation:** This is a powerful technique in combating stress. Mindful meditation can regulate cortisol. It can also help boost concentration and encourage a state of relaxation, leading to a happy and healthy life.

Taking Action: when to Seek Professional Help

Due to the adverse effects of poor mental health in your daily life, recognizing when to seek help is crucial in managing hormonal imbalances effectively. If symptoms are severe, significantly impacting your daily life, or not improving with lifestyle changes, it's time to seek professional help. Regular check-ups can help monitor hormonal health and catch imbalances early. Working with healthcare professionals who specialize in hormonal health, like endocrinologists or functional medicine practitioners, can ensure you get the right care.

Chapter Four

Unmasking Hormone Tests

Your Guide to Understanding Hormonal Check-ups

"*H*ormonal imbalances can cause many symptoms but that does not mean they are the cause of all your symptoms. So how can you tell when it's your hormones or something else?"
 – Pelin Batur, MD, women's health specialist

As a woman who has begun her menstrual cycle or is nearing menopause, you will go through a series of changes, both physically and mentally. It can be tempting to blame every symptom you experience on your hormones but they're not always the culprits.

So, first you need to identify if your hormones are the issue. Then, if the symptoms are a result of your hormones, the next step is to figure out which one is causing the problem. Is it estrogen, cortisol, testosterone, progesterone, or another kind of hormone? Lastly, could the symptoms you're experiencing be a result of your hormone levels being too high or too low?

Again, even though you may be experiencing symptoms of hormonal imbalance, it does not mean you *have* a hormonal imbalance. This is why hormonal testing is of great importance. Testing will enable you to take a deep dive into your symptoms individually so you can consider all the factors, whether it be lifestyle or an underlying medical condition.

Why Hormone Testing is Important

Hormone testing provides a snapshot of your hormonal health, enabling early intervention if imbalances are detected. Getting your hormones tested and analyzed is important if you are experiencing specific symptoms and health problems. It can also give you vital information about your health and well-being and how you can optimize and regulate your hormones to feel your best.

In the event that preliminary testing of your hormones uncovers an imbalance or concerning fluctuations, a personalized treatment plan can be established by your doctor—preferably a hormone health practitioner—based on your hormonal readings. Also, in order to achieve optimal hormone levels, continuous testing will be carried out to monitor the effectiveness of the treatment you will receive.

According to the Hormone Health Network, regular hormone testing can help identify imbalances that may be causing symptoms such as fatigue, mood swings, weight gain, and fertility issues, which are all common in women aged twenty to sixty.

For example, you may be experiencing chronic acne, which could mean you have increased levels of the male hormone androgen, particularly testosterone. Acne can also be a symptom of polycystic ovary syndrome (PCOS). Even thyroid imbalances can cause acne. It can be complex to figure out. With all these different hormones at play, you might assume your acne is a result of your hormones being out of sync, but it could also be related to stress, poor sleeping habits, a change in diet, bacteria, or inflammation.

Regular testing allows for tracking hormonal changes over time, providing critical insight into your body's response to lifestyle changes, nutritional shifts, or therapy.

Hormone levels can also vary widely among women. Tests provide personalized data, allowing you to understand your unique hormonal profile and tailor your wellness approach accordingly.

Different Types of Hormone Tests

Your hormone levels can be tested using saliva, urine, or blood samples. Deciding which type of hormone test to take will be based on your health, the hormones to be tested for, and if you're under any ongoing hormone treatments, among other factors, and they each come with their pros and cons.

- **Saliva hormone tests:** This is the simplest and least invasive hormone test when it comes to sample collection. It plays a crucial role in diagnosing and monitoring various health conditions. Saliva hormone testing involves analyzing the hormones present in your saliva to gain valuable information about how your endocrine system functions.

Compared to the total amount of hormones in your bloodstream, saliva tests provide an excellent picture of the active hormones available in your body. There are limitations to this type of testing, as some hormone concentrations can be higher or lower in saliva than in blood or urine.

Other factors taken into consideration with saliva testing include food intake, pH level in the mouth, the use of makeup, and teeth brushing.

Saliva testing primarily focuses on measuring steroid hormones like testosterone, cortisol, and DHEA-S (dehydroepiandrosterone). It also tests for the female sex hormones estrogen (all three types) and progesterone.

The process of saliva hormone testing starts with the collection of saliva samples at specific times of the day or over several days, as hormone levels can vary throughout the day. After collection, a laboratory can analyze combined samples or individual samples of saliva using advanced techniques like enzyme immunoassays (EIA) or radioimmunoassays (RIA) to determine the accurate measurements of hormone levels in the saliva.

- **Blood serum hormone tests:** Blood serum hormone tests involve the analysis of hormones present in the blood, useful in the determination of the concentration of specific hormones in your bloodstream to aid diagnosis and management of hormone disorders.

Blood serum tests analyze blood in its original form, unlike the blood spot test which stores blood in dried form until it's ready for use. This means the shelf-life of blood serum tests is slightly shorter. Blood serum samples are commonly collected through a vein in your arm, and to ensure accurate measurements, you may be required to fast before the time of the blood draw.

Although blood serum tests have a short shelf-life, they encompass a broad range of hormones for hormone testing. These hormones include:

- Thyroid hormones - Triiodothyronine (T3) and thyroxine(T4)

- Reproductive hormones (estrogen, progesterone, and testosterone)

- Insulin

- Cortisol

- Luteinizing hormone (LH)

- Follicle-stimulating hormone (FSH)

- Prolactin

- DHEA-S

- Prostate-specific antigen (PSA)

- Sex hormone-binding globulin (SHBG)

Blood Serum tests are a fundamental pillar in diagnosing endocrine disorders. For thyroid assessments, these tests aid in diagnosing hyperthyroidism, hypothyroidism, or thyroid dysfunction. In reproductive hormone profiling, blood serum tests aid in assessing fertility, menstrual irregularities, and reproductive health. Abnormality in insulin levels may indicate insulin resistance or diabetes mellitus, so blood tests have proven very effective in diabetes diagnosis.

Although these tests are quite versatile, they can be invasive and might not reflect hormone levels in tissues. Blood tests are not ideal for measuring hormone levels influenced by hormone replacement therapy (HRT) gels and other topical creams. HRT gels contain estradiol, which is identical to the naturally occurring estrogen, so blood tests to check your estradiol levels can be prone to error.

- **Urine hormone tests:** Urine tests serve as a window into your body's endocrine system by examining the level of various hormones excreted in urine. They offer a comprehensive view of hormone metabolites and are excellent for mapping out the full hormonal picture. Unlike blood serum tests, urine tests are non-invasive and offer an accessible means of assessing your hormones.

Hormones are circulated in the bloodstream by the endocrine glands, and eventually, they break down and form by-products, or metabolites, which are excreted through the kidneys into urine. To carry out this test, multiple samples of your urine will be collected at intervals over a specified period.

It could span from an hour to a 24-hour collection. The duration it takes depends on the specific hormone being assessed. Multiple samples allow for the provision of a comprehensive assessment, capturing all hormonal fluctuations and patterns that may be missed in single-point blood tests.

Urine tests allow medical practitioners to assess how the body metabolizes hormones, which serves as an opportunity to identify potential risks like cancer. These tests measure free hormones, including estrogen (estrone, estradiol, and estriol), testosterone, progesterone, cortisol, melatonin, and DHEA-S.

Unlike blood tests, urine tests are useful in patients using the topical form of hormone replacement therapy and are also capable of measuring more types of estrogen hormones than blood tests.

- **Blood spot testing:** This type of hormone test is minimally invasive. It requires pricking the finger with a needle to release blood. The blood is usually dropped in multiple spots on the filter card and left to dry.

The blood spot test method is limited in the variety of hormones it can test. It can be used to assess the following: insulin, thyroid hormones, estrogen (estradiol), DHEA-S, progesterone, testosterone, luteinizing hormone, and follicle-stimulating hormone. Blood spot tests produce accurate results for many critical hormones and are an effective way of monitoring hormone levels in people using hormone replacement therapy (HRT) gels or topical creams, unlike blood serum testing.

How to Interpret Hormone Test Results

If you suspect the symptoms you may be experiencing could be related to hormonal imbalance, getting your hormones tested is recommended. A hormone test enables you to understand the makeup of your hormones, meaning that you can quickly identify conditions that might arise before or after menopause, including thyroid disease and PCOS. This is key to taking appropriate action.

There are up to fifty hormones present in the body. A female hormone test examines the most important female hormones, checking for any imbalance in their current levels. Remember, when hormone levels are too high or too low, they can negatively impact your health.

The hormone levels obtained from the test results can tell your doctor a lot about the symptoms you may be experiencing, from fertility to constant fatigue, or unexplained weight gain or loss. It can help them catch and address a lot of issues on time. Women over forty are advised to go for hormone tests because, during this period, their bodies and hormones will go through a series of drastic changes as a result of menopause.

A female hormonal profile assesses the following hormones in your body:

- Estrogen (Estradiol)

- Progesterone

- Follicle-stimulating hormone (FSH)

- Testosterone

- Thyroid hormones

Test results

To check that there are no irregularities, your hormone levels will be compared with normal, or reference, values. Test results typically provide reference ranges, but it's important to remember these ranges represent averages and may not be optimal for every individual.

Results should be interpreted in the context of your symptoms. For example, you might have normal estrogen levels, but if you're experiencing symptoms of estrogen dominance, you may need to consider other factors like progesterone levels or liver health.

- **Estrogen blood test:** Estrogen is the female sex hormone responsible for developing and regulating secondary sex characteristics in women. Your hormone tests will normally check for estradiol, as it's the most active and potent form of estrogen in your body.

Estradiol plays a vital role in pregnancy, ovulation, skin and bone health, and many more areas, but as you reach menopause, the levels of this hormone begin to decline.

At the beginning of your cycle, estradiol levels range between 27 pg/ml to 161 pg/ml. In a fertile woman, the level should be below 50 pg/ml. High estradiol levels are associated with symptoms like obesity and issues with sex drive and fatigue, while low levels can mean PCOS, poor ovarian reserve, low libido, anorexia, or a decrease in pituitary function.

- **Progesterone tests:** Serum progesterone, as it is normally called on a blood test, is a test to measure the amount of progesterone in the blood. Progesterone levels vary, depending on when it is done during your cycle. Normal progesterone levels on day twenty-one of your cycle must range below 5 and 20 ng/l, preferably 10ng/ml or below to confirm ovulation has happened.

On the third day of your cycle, they should be lower than 1.5 ng/ml, and in postmenopausal women, they are less than 1 ng/ml. High progesterone is associated with symptoms like anxiety, depression, reduced libido, and weight fluctuations, while low levels of progesterone can result in irregular menstrual periods, headaches, and spotting.

- **Follicle-stimulating hormone tests:** The follicle-stimulating hormone is in charge of the menstrual cycle in women and dictates when ovaries produce eggs. During your cycle, FSH levels vary and are usually at a peak immediately before ovulation.

It's important to have this hormone tested as it helps diagnose the start of menopause, as well as ovarian issues like cysts, infertility, and abnormal menstrual bleeding. Levels between 3 to 9 mlU/ml are signs of a good ovarian reserve. A value below 6 indicates that the ovarian reserve is excellent. From 6 to 9, it's good, between 9 to 10 moderate, and 10-13 indicates a diminished egg count. Values above 13 mIU/ml show a very low ovarian reserve, which typically occurs when menopause starts.

- **Testosterone tests:** Normal testosterone levels in women lie between 24 and 47 ng/dl. Elevated levels are usually an indicator of PCOS, but can also indicate ovarian cancer or cancer of the adrenal glands. Your testosterone levels will typically drop during menopause, which can lead to issues such as depression and loss of sex drive.

- **Thyroid tests:** Levels of triiodothyronine (T3) on day three of your cycle should range between approximately 1.4 and 4.4 pg/ml, while thyroxine (T4) should be between 0.8 and 2 ng/dl.

All these concepts may be a bit complex for you to understand, And that's why it's necessary to consult a knowledgeable healthcare professional who can properly interpret test results and develop a plan of action. A functional medicine practitioner can provide insights not only on the numbers but also on the root cause of imbalances.

When to Seek Professional Help

Professional guidance is crucial in managing hormonal health effectively. Consulting a healthcare professional is advised if your test results show significant hormonal imbalances or if you're experiencing severe symptoms.

For complex conditions like PCOS or endometriosis, a specialist's guidance can be invaluable in navigating the condition and devising a comprehensive management plan.

Regular check-ups with a healthcare professional can help monitor progress and adjust your wellness plan as necessary. For example, a nutritional tweak might be needed if an initial approach doesn't improve symptoms of hormonal imbalance.

The Future of Hormone Testing

Advancements in technology are making hormone testing more accessible and personalized. At-home hormone testing kits, like those offered by companies such as EverlyWell and LetsGetChecked, are making it easier to monitor hormonal health from the comfort of your home. These tests typically involve simple procedures, like finger pricks for blood tests or saliva collection, and the samples are sent to a lab for analysis.

While these tests should not replace professional healthcare advice, they can provide useful initial insights and stimulate more informed conversations with healthcare providers.

CHAPTER FIVE

Nourishing Your Hormones

A Deep Dive into Nutritional Balance

"*Food is medicine, and the right kind of relationship with food can make a positive impact on your health.*"
– Hayley Hobson, Certified Life and Health Coach

These wise words from holistic health practitioner Hayley Hobson emphasize the pivotal role food plays in your health and wellness. Nutrition and dietary patterns can either prove beneficial or detrimental to your hormonal balance in the long run. I'll tell you why.

Ever heard the phrase "food is fuel"? It's a common saying, but what does it mean? Well, think of the body as a vehicle. Vehicles require petrol or diesel to function and move from one place to another. And like these vehicles, our bodies require fuel to function. In our case, we need food. And, if our bodies are going to function effectively and efficiently, we can't just eat any food; we need a well-balanced diet.

So you might ask, "How does food affect our hormones?" Food provides the energy and nutrients required to fuel your body. If we do not eat food with the nutrients the body needs, our bodies can fail to produce hormones correctly. This can cause our hormonal balance to suffer because the body lacks the basic building blocks to attain equilibrium. That's why this chapter explores the pivotal role of nutritional balance in hormonal health. We will take a deep dive on how to eat for hormonal balance, as well as taking a look at foods to avoid in order to maintain hormonal balance. We will also explore highly nutritious and tasty meal plans and recipes that will help you achieve and keep a restored and balanced hormonal system.

The Plate and Your Hormones: Understanding the Connection

Nutrition is more than just fuel; it's a key player in hormonal balance. What we eat can significantly impact hormone production and function because key nutrients in these foods help to keep our endocrine system healthy and impact circulating levels of certain hormones.

For example, consuming a diet with too much sugar and refined carbohydrates can lead to insulin resistance (a common hormone issue), type 2 diabetes, hypertension, and cardiovascular disease. Insulin, a hormone produced by the pancreas, regulates blood sugar levels. When we consistently consume high-sugar foods, our body's need for insulin increases, which can eventually lead to insulin resistance.

Did you know that some of the most active hormones in the body are synthesized from cholesterol? Steroid hormones, which include testosterone, progesterone, and estrogen, all need cholesterol.

According to Dr. Ghazala Aziz-Scott, a hormone specialist at the Marion Gluck Clinic, high levels of cholesterol are quite infamous for causing cholesterol plaque buildup, furring the arteries, and leading to heart diseases.

However, cholesterol does not only pose negative effects for the body. It can also have a positive impact, depending on its levels in the body. For example, women with extremely low body fat are prone to suffering from the absence of their menstrual periods (amenorrhea) and infertility. This is due to a level of cholesterol in the body that is insufficient for synthesizing estrogen and progesterone, which are essential female sex hormones in the reproductive system.

Another example can be seen in the case of excessive intake of red meat, which can increase the production of estrogen in your body. Studies show that when estrogen levels are too high, they can result in reproductive health problems like polycystic ovary syndrome, painful periods, fibroids, and increased endometriosis pain.

On the flip side, eating a balanced diet rich in lean proteins, healthy fats, and a variety of fruits and vegetables can help maintain hormonal balance. These foods provide the essential nutrients our bodies need to produce and regulate hormones effectively.

Certain nutrients are particularly important for hormone health. For instance, omega-3 fatty acids—found in fatty fish like salmon—play a critical role in producing hormones, reducing inflammation, and may help regulate menstrual cycles in women with polycystic ovary syndrome (PCOS).

Vitamin D, often referred to as the sunshine vitamin, plays a crucial role in hormone production, including insulin and thyroid hormones. It's found in foods like fatty fish, cheese, and egg yolks, but can also be obtained through sun exposure.

Magnesium—found in foods like almonds, black beans, and spinach—is essential for many processes in the body, including regulating the nervous system and improving insulin sensitivity.

Food Friends and Foes: What to Embrace and What to Avoid

Understanding nutrition-hormone relationships is a key part of the functional and holistic medicine approach to hormonal balance. Not all foods are created equal when it comes to hormonal health. Some foods are hormone heroes, while others can disrupt your hormonal harmony.

Maintaining a sustainable diet filled with nutritious and unprocessed food is the goal here. There are certain foods commonly labeled as "good," such as grains, fruits, and vegetables. But too much of anything is bad, even the good ones, as it's still possible to over consume these good foods.

This is why it's highly important to eat a well-balanced and diverse meal. It ensures your body and its hormones get the nourishment they require to carry out their respective functions.

I curated an ideal hormone-balancing plate of the food groups your meals should consist of. The ones that are highly recommended for balancing and sustaining your hormones. Your hormone-balancing plate should consist of about 40 percent vegetables (cruciferous vegetables included), 10 percent healthy fats, 20 percent lean protein, and 30 percent whole grains.

It may be difficult to get your percentages right; however, you should aim to incorporate a portion of each food group into your meals every day.

Foods to Embrace for Hormonal Balance

- **Cruciferous vegetables:** These are green vegetables that belong to the edible cabbage family, genus *Brassica*. They include leafy greens, broccoli, brussels sprouts, cauliflower, radishes, turnips, kale, arugula, cabbage, and many more.

Cruciferous vegetables contain compounds that help detoxify estrogen. They have proven beneficial to women with conditions like estrogen dominance, where estrogen levels are much higher than levels of progesterone in the body.

These vegetables are rich in nutrients. They include several vitamins, like vitamin C, K, and E. They're also a good source of fiber, which helps lower estrogen levels. You can include these green leafy vegetables in your daily diet, but remember, balance is key. Too much of these vegetables can cause thyroid damage, especially for people with thyroid problems.

- **Fish:** Fatty fish—like salmon, mackerel, black cod, and tuna—are excellent sources of omega-3 fatty acids. These essential fats help regulate hormone levels, reduce menstrual pain, and also support healthy fetal development during pregnancy. Fish is also rich in vitamin D and selenium, vitamins that help support thyroid hormone production.

- **Flaxseeds:** These are a type of phytoestrogen that help balance estrogen levels in the body. Phytoestrogens are plant-derived compounds, and they behave similarly to estrogen. Foods rich in phytoestrogens, like flaxseed, help to reduce hot flashes and other perimenopausal symptoms, relieve menstrual issues or irregularities, and relieve or prevent acne. Other sources of phytoestrogens include oats, yams, beans, legumes, carrots, and apples.

- **Quinoa:** When you eat carbohydrates with a high glycemic index, such as white rice, white bread, sugary foods, and most breakfast cereals, they break down and get absorbed easily in the body. The glucose from these carbs travels through your bloodstream, signaling the pancreas to produce insulin. Eating too many calories from these foods can make you gain weight, increase your risk of insulin resistance, and make you more likely to suffer from diabetes. These spikes in blood sugar levels may also result in hormonal imbalance.

Quinoa is a healthy alternative to these foods. It has a low glycemic index and can help promote hormone health by controlling sugar levels in the blood. Quinoa also helps reduce belly fat and may improve PCOS symptoms.

- **Avocados:** These fruits are high in antioxidants and rich in healthy fats and fiber. They contain compounds that help control insulin levels, boost your metabolism, limit the secretion of the stress hormone cortisol, and improve muscle functionality. In cases where the body secretes excess estrogen, avocados possess the ability to block estrogen absorption, in turn boosting the levels of progesterone in women.

Excess estrogen can be caused by exposure to toxic pollutants in the environment, hormones from food, and chemical estrogens in plastics. Introducing avocado to your daily diet helps to soften the toxic load and balance your hormones effectively.

- **Eggs:** Eggs are a great source of protein and are one of the best foods out there for hormonal balance. They are a great source of HDL cholesterol, which is the healthy type of cholesterol required by the body to produce hormones. Eggs are also nutrient-rich in vitamin D and vitamin B6, which are beneficial for estrogen metabolism.

They also have a positive impact on the insulin and ghrelin hormones in the body. Insulin controls blood sugar levels, while ghrelin's primary function is to control appetite. It has been observed that insulin and ghrelin levels are lower after eating eggs for breakfast.

Foods to Avoid when Reducing Hormonal Imbalance

It's essential to know that not all foods are beneficial to your health. Certain foods can negatively affect hormone levels in the body. It's important to be aware of these foods, as they can lead to future health problems simply by causing an upward spike or a decline in your hormones.

- **Sugary foods and beverages:** Consuming sugary foods and beverages can significantly impact your hormonal system. When you eat sugary foods—like cakes, chocolates, candies, and soft drinks—they can gradually reduce the sensitivity of the hormones leptin and ghrelin, which regulate appetite and indicate fullness.

Indulging in these high-sugar items, especially refined sugars, tends to trigger a spike in blood sugar levels. In response, the pancreas secretes insulin to regulate this urge. Consistent consumption of sugary foods can result in insulin resistance. Too much insulin can cause a drop in a crucial protein that helps regulate the levels of testosterone the body can use, called sex hormone-binding globulin (SHBG), disrupting the intricate balance of hormone regulation.

- **Alcohol:** The liver is vital in regulating balance in sex hormones, thyroid hormones, and various adrenal hormones. Excessive consumption of alcohol can affect the liver. Another notable effect alcohol intake has on the body is the stress hormone cortisol. Moderate consumption of alcohol can temporarily reduce cortisol levels, but excessive drinking can lead to an increase in cortisol levels.

- **Excessive red meat:** Red meat can influence hormonal health, primarily due to its high content of saturated fats. Diets rich in saturated fats have been associated with increased levels of insulin resistance. Eating a lot of red meat can cause an increase in estrogen levels, and when estrogen levels are very high, it can result in reproductive health problems like PCOS, fibroids, and painful periods.

- **Processed foods:** Processed foods can exert detrimental effects on hormonal health due to their often high levels of added sugars, salt, unhealthy fats, and artificial preservatives. These ingredients can lead to inflammation and stress in your adrenal glands, which may lead to weight gain or contribute to deficiencies that can impact overall endocrine health. Avoiding these foods or consuming them in moderation is advisable.

- **Caffeine:** This is a nervous system stimulant, and it's mostly found in coffee, tea, and various sodas or energy drinks. When consumed in moderation, it can enhance the release of adrenaline, which supports short-term energy bursts and increased alertness. However, high doses of caffeine in the system can stimulate the release of more cortisol, potentially contributing to elevated stress levels. Prolonged elevation of these stress hormones can interfere with sleep patterns, causing you to feel fatigued, irritable, or anxious during the day.

- **Carbohydrates with a high glycemic index:** As we discussed, foods with a high glycemic index are easily digested and absorbed into the body, causing a spike in blood sugar levels. When your blood sugar goes up very fast, it tends to interfere with hormones like insulin, as the abrupt rise and fall in blood sugar levels prompts an insulin surge to move glucose into cells and tissues. Over time, it can contribute to insulin resistance.

Meal Planning for Hormonal Health: Practical Tips and Recipes

Having a plan is key to maintaining a hormone-friendly diet. Meal planning can take the stress out of eating healthy and ensure you're providing your body with the nutrients it needs to maintain hormonal balance.

Try to include a good balance of macronutrients (proteins, fats, and carbs) at each meal. For example, a dinner could include grilled salmon (protein and healthy fats), quinoa (complex carbs), and a side of broccoli and bell peppers (vegetables and fiber).

Snacks can also be hormone-healthy. Try almond butter on whole grain toast or a smoothie with spinach, frozen berries, flax seeds, and unsweetened almond milk.

Recipes can be simple, tasty, and hormone-friendly. If you are stuck for ideas on what to eat for hormone balancing, here are a couple of examples:

- **Hormone-balancing breakfast bowl:** Start your day with a bowl of cooked quinoa, topped with a hard-boiled egg, avocado slices, and a sprinkle of chia seeds. This meal packs protein, healthy fats, and fiber to keep your hormones happy.

- **Soothing turmeric tea:** Turmeric is known for its anti-inflammatory properties. Brew a cup of warm turmeric tea with almond milk, honey, and a pinch of black pepper (which helps your body absorb the beneficial compound in turmeric called curcumin). Sip this in the evening to wind down your day and support your hormones.

- **Zingy salmon and cauliflower salad:** Have you ever considered a delicious salmon and cauliflower salad for a hormone-friendly meal? Salmon is a fatty fish loaded with omega-3 fatty acids. Omega-3 fats are known for making hormones that regulate blood clotting and inflammation, keeping everything ship-shape. Cauliflower, on the other hand, is rich in fiber and antioxidants and contains compounds known to detoxify estrogen. Eaten together with salmon, it makes a dynamic duo. To give the salmon a zingy kick, try marinating it in a mixture of fresh lemon juice, minced garlic, and dill. The bright citrus flavors pair beautifully with the rich salmon, while the garlic and dill add an aromatic punch. Grill or bake the marinated salmon until it's perfectly flaky and tender.

For the salad base, roast some cauliflower florets with a drizzle of olive oil, salt, and pepper until they're slightly charred and crispy. Toss the roasted cauliflower with mixed greens, cherry tomatoes, sliced cucumber, and red onion for a fresh and crunchy base.

Top the salad with the zingy salmon, and finish it off with a sprinkle of toasted almonds or pumpkin seeds for an added crunch. A light vinaigrette made with olive oil, lemon juice, and Dijon mustard would be the perfect dressing to tie all the flavors together.

This power-packed salad is not only hormone-friendly but also a nutritional powerhouse, providing a perfect balance of lean protein, healthy fats, fiber, and antioxidants. Enjoy it as a satisfying lunch or a light dinner, and feel the goodness nourishing your body from the inside out.

- **Roasted bacon brussels sprouts with salted honey:** Not only does this combo sound mouth-watering, it also works wonders for your hormones. Brussels sprouts are loaded with a ton of nutrients, which have been shown to reduce high estrogen levels. For flavor, add a dash of crispy bacon and drizzle some salted honey for a touch of natural sweetness.

- **Salmon salad with beets, arugula, pistachios, and pomegranates:** This dish is loaded with so many healthy yet tasty ingredients. It's perfect for lunch or dinner and can be ready in under thirty minutes. Salmon brings its A-game with omega-3 fatty acids, and beets rich in antioxidants add that pop of color to the meal. Let's not forget the pistachios, arugula, and pomegranates, which are packed with healthy fats and antioxidants and add a sweet-tart flair to your deliciously balanced meal.

- **Chocolate chia pudding:** This meal is a nutritious way to start your morning. Chia seeds are packed with omega-3 fatty acids and fiber, and they work wonders at contributing to hormonal balance. Dark chocolate, rich in antioxidants, is used for the pudding. And guess what? It's super easy to whip up. Indulge in this nourishing treat, and your taste buds and hormones will thank you.

Share Your Light

As women, we possess an incredible inner light that guides us through the complexities of life. By sharing our experiences and insights, we can illuminate the path for others on a similar journey. That's why I'm humbly asking you to consider leaving a review for "Understanding Hormones for Women" – not for personal gain, but to empower and inspire fellow seekers of holistic wellness.

Your review, no matter how brief, can be a beacon of hope for someone navigating the intricate world of hormones and overall well-being. It's a simple act of generosity that costs you nothing but a few moments of your time, yet it holds the potential to profoundly impact countless lives.

Imagine a woman, much like yourself, seeking guidance on her path to balance and vitality. Your honest words could be the nudge she needs to embark on a transformative journey, one that empowers her to embrace her unique feminine essence and unlock a newfound sense of harmony within.

To leave a review, simply visit the book's page on Amazon and share your authentic experience. Your words, born from a place of compassion and understanding, will resonate deeply with those seeking the same wisdom you have gained.

Scan here for the review page!

Remember, by sharing our light, we create a ripple effect that extends far beyond our individual journeys. Together, we can illuminate the path for countless women, guiding them towards a life of balance, vitality, and profound self-discovery.

Thank you for considering this humble request. Your thoughtful review is a gift that will continue to give, empowering women to embrace their innate strength and reclaim their well-being.

With heartfelt gratitude,
Dr. Ashley Sullivan, PharmD

Chapter Six

Herbs at Your Service

Natural Allies for Hormonal Balance

Did you know that herbal remedies and plant medicines were among the first and only medicines to be used throughout all of human history? Until the mid-nineteenth century when human beings began to develop synthetic medicines. Prior to this time, natural substances were used to make effective natural remedies.

Despite the development of more researched orthodox medicines, herbal remedies continue to be well-patronized by people across the world. This comes from the belief that orthodox medicines give "quick" relief while herbal remedies give "total" healing.

Although the general public has come to rely on orthodox medicine greatly, medication and surgery seldom address the root causes of diseases or, in this case, hormone imbalances. Many female problems can be helped with simple herbs for self-treatment at home, certain

UNDERSTANDING LEAKY GUT & HORMONES... 257

lifestyle changes, and diet. Herbs are safe, well-tolerated by the body, super affordable to purchase, and can easily be grown in your backyard. Some herbs, however, are potent and should be taken with the same level of caution as pharmaceutical medications. It's important to properly identify these herbs and purchase them from a reputable su pplier.

As we delve deeper into this chapter, I will pass along my knowledge on various herbs and natural supplements to support hormonal balance. I will also provide practical advice on their safe and effective use, and together, we will learn more about the use of herbs for natural remedies so that you can regain the control you need over your health.

Harnessing the Power of Herbal Allies

A study was carried out to investigate the efficacy of the woodland herb, black cohosh, on the reduction of vasomotor symptoms (cardinal symptoms of menopause like hot flashes and night sweats) in women aged fifty to fifty-nine. It was observed that black cohosh proved beneficial in reducing the frequency of vasomotor symptoms. Preparations that contained black cohosh improved symptoms overall by 26 percent, while trials that combined black cohosh with other products improved symptoms by 41 percent (Shams 2010).

In another study carried out on early postmenopausal Caucasian women to check the hormone-balancing effect of pre-gelatinized organic Maca (*Lepidium peruvianum* Chacon), Maca was found to significantly stimulate the production of estradiol (E2) in women who met the criteria, with simultaneous suppression of follicle-stimulating hormone (Meissner 2006). Menopausal symptoms were assessed according to Greene's Score (GMS) and Kupperman's Index (KMI), which are commonly used in clinical studies to determine menopausal symptom prevalence.

Upon conclusion of this study, organic Maca (Maca-GO) was found to significantly reduce both frequency and severity of individual menopausal symptoms (hot flushes and night sweating in particular). It offers an attractive non-hormonal addition to the choices available to early-postmenopausal women, allowing them to reduce their dependence on hormone therapy programs, such as Hormone Replacement Therapy (HRT).

There is a lot of overlap between hormonal balance and herbal benefits, and in the next section, I will walk you through them.

Herbs That Support Hormonal Balance

From time immemorial, the knowledge of herbal remedies has been passed down through generations, forming the cornerstone of women's healthcare. Whether it be relieving menstrual pain or irregularities, supporting fertility, or easing the transition through menopause, herbs have played a vital role in promoting hormonal harmony. Some of the herbs that are still commonly used in herbal medicine to balance hormones naturally include:

- **Chaste Tree Berry (Vitex agnus-castus):** This fantastic herb is native to the Mediterranean region and has a long history of supporting women's hormonal health. The plant is known to help balance the production levels of hormones like prolactin, progesterone, and estrogen by acting on the pituitary gland, which plays a key role for women with irregular periods.

A study in the journal *Planta Medica* found that the chaste tree reduced symptoms of premenstrual syndrome. The herb is often employed to alleviate symptoms associated with premenstrual syndrome (PMS), such as mood swings, bloating, and breast tenderness.

Moreover, it may support fertility by promoting a more regular ovulation pattern. Many women have found relief from hormonal imbalances with the regular use of the chaste tree berry or its supplements.

Some women may experience some side effects like skin reactions or gastrointestinal discomfort, but not to worry, if there are side effects, they are usually mild. However, as with any herbal remedy, consulting with a healthcare professional or a qualified medical herbalist is important.

You can find local qualified herbalists through the National Institute of Medical Herbalists or the College of Practitioners of Phytotherapy.

- **Black Cohosh (Actaea racemosa):** This herb is a traditional Native American remedy for menopausal symptoms. It has gained popularity and a lot of scientific attention for its effects on hot flashes and mood swings.

Black cohosh works in the thalamus, supporting hormonal balance during menopause and body temperature regulation. A review in Obstetrics and Gynecology International found it to be effective and safe. Although studies of its effectiveness in reducing hot flashes have produced mixed results, some women report that it has greatly helped them.

While it is safe for consumption, excess consumption of black cohosh may lead to headaches or gastrointestinal disturbances, with some reports linking it to liver problems.

- **Dong Quai (Angelica sinensis):** This is a renowned herb deeply rooted in traditional Chinese medicine. Often referred to as the female ginseng, or the women's herb, it's one of the most used herbs and has been traditionally used to address a spectrum of women's health issues, particularly those related to the reproductive system, for more than 1,200 years.

This herb helps moderate the production of the hormone estrogen in the body and may increase its production. It can also help alleviate menstrual and menopausal symptoms like cramps, night sweats, migraines, and many more. After childbirth, dong quai can be administered to ease tiredness and aid in speedy recovery for women.

It can also be taken to promote fertility in some women. Not only does Dong quai help in balancing hormones, but it also possesses the ability to help balance body sugar, beautify and speed up healing of the skin, reduce inflammation, regulate the immune system, and promote proper circulation in the body.

Dong quai should never be used by women with fibroids or blood-clotting problems such as hemophilia, or by some women with hormone-sensitive cancers, due to the adverse effects of having high estrogen levels in the body.

- **Maca (Lepidium meyenii):** This is a root vegetable found in South America, particularly Peru and Bolivia. The Maca plant is a cruciferous vegetable, like cauliflower and brussels sprouts. It's also rich in vitamins like C, A, B2, and many more.

Maca has gained significant recognition for its positive impact on women's hormones. It can be classified as a herbal adaptogen, meaning that it can directly change the balance of your hormones to help you adapt to stress and illness.

Your endocrine system is at the forefront when it comes to handling the effects of stress or anxiety on your body, so the adaptogen effects of Maca help your endocrine system, causing it to lessen some of that load.

Maca helps prevent adrenal exhaustion, which occurs when your hormones are out of balance, causing constant tiredness and burnout, and it also helps in supporting your body's production of various hormones, alternating their levels, depending on what you need.

Moving on to women going through perimenopause and menopause, Maca can serve as a sort of hormone replacement therapy. Unlike some herbs that try to mimic estrogen in the body, Maca tends to increase the body's production of estrogen (estradiol), if the levels present are too low. Also, in peri- and menopausal women, Maca has been found to cause an increase in the levels of some hormones like progesterone and luteinizing hormone—both of which stimulate ovary function.

The stress hormone, cortisol, has also been proven to be suppressed upon consumption of Maca. Some women report improvements in energy levels, mood, and libido with reductions in hot flashes, night sweats, insomnia, and depression.

While considered generally safe, individual responses to this herb may vary. Women with overactive thyroid issues may experience side effects on consumption. Hence, it's advisable to consult with a healthcare professional before embracing Maca as a holistic addition to your health and wellness.

- **Red clover (Trifolium pratense):** This herb contains phytoestrogens, particularly isoflavones, which partially mimic the action of estrogen in the body. Although phytoestrogens are known to mimic naturally occurring estrogen, they are not identical to the original. But they can still bind to estrogen receptors and influence hormones.

Traditionally used by the Native Americans for treating whooping cough, gout, and cancer, red clover has been found to decrease the vasomotor symptoms of menopause, such as hot flashes and mood swings, due to its ability to interact with estrogen receptors.

In women who have had estrogen-receptor-positive cancer, the use of red clover is strongly advised against, as the herb can stimulate an increase in estrogen-positive cancer cells. Red clover has also been identified as containing compounds that can cause the blood to thin, and as a result, patients on anticoagulants such as aspirin, Coumadin, and heparin should be dissuaded from using this herb because it may put them at an increased risk of bleeding.

- **Lady's mantle (Alchemilla vulgaris):** This is such an interesting name for an herb, and it has proven itself to be a woman's best friend. Native to Europe and Asia, the lady's mantle helps in relieving painful and heavy periods, menopausal symptoms, as well as gastrointestinal issues like diarrhea.

Lady's mantle stimulates the production of progesterone resulting in a regular menstrual period. Low levels of progesterone tend to cause abnormality in ovulation patterns and irregular menstruation, which could lead to infertility problems in the future. This herb combats fertility problems, too.

It's favored due to its ability to soothe menstrual pain and even make your flow lighter. The lady's mantle is able to subdue excessive menstrual flow, as in the case of menorrhagia, and also regulate irregular menstrual bleeding, in cases of metrorrhagia. Another benefit of this herb is that it can tone and tighten the skin, giving a luminous, glowing, and healthy complexion.

You can consume Lady's Mantle in a variety of forms. However, some herbalists recommend taking it in its tea form, especially when it's being used to help women prepare and recover from childbirth.

Incorporating one or more of these herbs for hormonal balance into your lifestyle can help you on your journey to achieving hormonal balance and becoming a better and healthier you. It's important to remember that herbs are potent and should be used with caution. Always consult with a healthcare professional before starting any new supplement regimen.

Moreover, herbs can interact with medications you're already taking, so it's important to provide your doctor with a complete list of all the supplements you're using. Remember, it's also crucial to purchase supplements from reputable sources to ensure quality and safety. Companies like Gaia Herbs and Mountain Rose Herbs are known for their rigorous testing and high-quality products.

Over-the-Counter Supplements for Hormonal Health

Certain over-the-counter (OTC) supplements can also support hormonal balance. It's important to choose quality supplements and use them as directed for the best results.

- **Omega-3 Fatty Acids:** These essential fats are known to support hormonal health. A study in the Journal of Clinical Endocrinology and Metabolism linked omega-3 supplementation with improved hormonal balance in women with polycystic ovary syndrome (PCOS).

- **Probiotics:** These beneficial bacteria support gut health, which in turn supports hormonal balance. The Journal of Functional Foods published a study showing that probiotics could help reduce symptoms of PCOS.

- **Magnesium:** This essential mineral can help with hormonal symptoms like PMS and sleep disturbances. The Journal of Women's Health reported that magnesium reduced PMS symptoms in women.

- **Ashwagandha:** This natural remedy for hormonal balance has proven effective in boosting thyroid function and balancing adrenal hormones and androgens. Not only does this herb help bring hormones back into balance, but it also boosts libido, increases energy levels, reduces inflammation, prevents depression, and balances blood sugar levels.

- **Zinc:** This mineral is required for thyroid hormone balance as a deficiency in zinc could result in symptoms of hypothyroidism. It also acts as an adaptogen, helping to rebalance excesses for various other hormones like progesterone, estrogen, and cortisol.

- **B vitamins:** These nutrients are essential for many bodily functions. They play a vital role in hormonal health as they are used as cofactors in detoxification. There are multiple B vitamins ranging from B-1 to B-12. But for this book, we will only emphasize the most beneficial B vitamins for your hormones.

- **Vitamin B3:** Also known as Niacin, B3 contributes to the production of sex hormones, including estrogen and progesterone, as well as stress (adrenal) hormones. Niacin also helps prevent inflammation.

- **Vitamin B6:** Also called pyrodoxine, B6 helps alleviate some premenstrual symptoms, like irritability and mood changes. It also helps the body effectively cope with stress, as it is a building block of the feel-good hormone, serotonin, as well as norepinephrine. Deficiencies in this vitamin can result in imbalances in the sex hormones, estrogen and progesterone. Taking supplements rich in vitamin B6 may also help with perimenopausal and menopausal symptoms in women.

- **Vitamin B12:** Cobalamin is essential for female reproductive health and pregnancy. Good levels of vitamin B12 have been found to maintain ovarian health. This vitamin also serves as a great detoxifier in the body and is very effective in balancing hormones in women's bodies.

The variety of B vitamins' important roles in the body mean that it's of great importance to consume enough of these nutrients, and in ways that allow them to be properly digested.

Supplements to Avoid Due to Potential Health Risks

In most cases, these multivitamins are not likely to pose risks to your health. However, it's important to be cautious, as some of these supplements can interact with other medications or pose risks if you have certain medical conditions like liver disease. Some of these supplements include:

- Gingko, which can increase the rate of blood thinning.

- St. John's wort, which can make some drugs like birth control lose some of their effectiveness.

- Herbal supplements like kava, which can cause damage to your liver.

- Vitamin A, which can increase the risk of lung cancer in smokers.

As with herbs, it's important to choose high-quality supplements from reputable companies. Look for products that have been independently tested for quality and purity. Companies like Thorne Research, NOW Foods, and Garden of Life are known for their high-quality supplements. It's also important to follow the dosage recommendations on the product label, as taking too much of a supplement can be harmful.

Navigating the World of Herbal Remedies and Supplements

Understanding how to navigate the world of herbal remedies and supplements can feel overwhelming, but with the right knowledge, you can make informed decisions that support your hormonal health. It's important to remember that everyone is unique, and what works for one person may not work for another. It may take some trial and error to find the right supplement regimen for you.

Keep in mind that supplements are just one piece of the puzzle. They should be used in conjunction with a healthy diet, regular exercise, and stress management techniques for the best results.

And finally, remember that achieving hormonal balance takes time. Be patient with yourself and celebrate every step forward on your journey to better health.

Chapter Seven

Balancing Act

Lifestyle Adjustments for Hormonal Harmony

"Take care of your body. It's the only place you have to live."
-Jim Rohn

Have you ever wondered about the intricate connection between your lifestyle habits and your hormonal balance? Naturally, your body produces the exact amount of hormones required to carry out various processes in the body.

However, due to certain factors like aging, sedentary lifestyles, dietary patterns, and other external factors beyond a person's control, your hormonal environment is bound to be affected. For many people, making small and simple lifestyle changes can help restore balance to the hormone levels in the body.

Jim Rohn's wise words echo this sentiment: "Our body is our only abode, and taking care of it is not just a choice but a responsibility.

Nurturing our bodies is paramount, and it's achieved through the daily choices we make."

In this chapter, we will delve into the world of hormones, where lifestyle habits like sleep, exercise, stress management, and gut health play a major role in shaping the melody of our overall well-being. As we embark on this journey, I will provide practical and actionable advice that you can incorporate into your everyday lives.

First, embracing quality sleep sets the stage for hormonal harmony. Imagine your hormonal harmony as a dazzling Broadway production where each component takes center stage. Sleep, in this grand spectacle, plays the role of the main act—a captivating performance that sets the tone for the entire show. It's not just about catching nightly shut-eye, but about a rejuvenating process that proves essential in maintaining balance in the hormones.

Now, let's talk about the transformative power of exercise and acknowledge its impact on your hormonal health. Boosting your physical activity can enhance your quality of life and help regulate hormonal imbalances.

Exercise is not just about sweating it out; it allows your body to embrace a state of balance and resilience. As a key player in the harmony of hormonal health, exercise serves as a productive outlet, stimulating the release of feel-good transmitters that help boost overall well-being.

Next up, stress management: In modern society, stress often plays an overpowering role that can disrupt the delicate balance of hormones. Navigating the journey of stress management would require us to unravel the impact of chronic stress on hormonal health, look at effective stress management techniques to support hormonal balance, and see the importance of seeking help when you feel overwhelmed.

Last but by no means least, gut health is central to your overall well-being, playing a large role in hormonal health. Beyond digestion, the gut influences far more than you realize. We will look at how your gut health affects your hormonal balance, ways you can improve your gut health, and when to seek help with gut issues.

Slumber Secrets: the Role of Sleep in Hormonal Health

In modern society, sleep has often been overlooked in the hustle and bustle of daily life. But it needs to be prioritized because it's a huge cornerstone of health and overall well-being due to the role it plays in hormonal health. Sleep is fundamental to hormonal balance, as it's during sleep that our bodies produce and regulate many hormones.

But before we take a deep dive into the profound influence sleep wields on our hormones, understanding what sleep is and why it's so important is pivotal. Appreciating the multifaceted nature of sleep lays the foundation for comprehending the profound influence it exerts on our hormonal health.

What Is Sleep, and Why Is It Important?

Sleep is a state in which consciousness is lost, and rousing the sleeper becomes increasingly difficult due to diminished motor function and sensory stimuli. It can be dissected into distinct categories. Namely, rapid eye movement (REM) and non-rapid eye movement (NREM) sleep.

Understanding these categories reveals the significance of a good night's sleep. Non-REM sleep serves as the foundation for restorative sleep and can be classified into three further phases: N1, N2, and N3, with N3 being the deepest.

The first phase (N1) marks the shift from wakefulness to sleep. It's the stage you enter when you gradually start nodding off, with your heartbeat, breathing activity, eye movements, and even brain waves slowing down.

The second phase (N2) brings about a deeper, continued state of the first phase, with limited awareness. During this phase, you are likely to experience a drop in body temperature and a further slowing of brain waves with occasional short bursts of brain activity, called sleep spindles, lasting for about 0.5 to 3 seconds.

The third phase (N3), also known as the deep sleep phase, is believed to be the most important phase for body and brain regeneration. Deep sleep helps regulate hormone release and glucose metabolism, among many other essential physiological processes crucial for overall health and well-being.

REM sleep, on the other hand, is marked by heightened brain activity and rapid eye movements. It occurs about ninety minutes after falling asleep and accounts for approximately 25 percent of your total time asleep. This stage of sleep is associated with vivid dreams, and it plays a significant role in impacting your memory, mood regulation, and improving mental focus.

Why Do We Need Sleep?

Prioritizing adequate sleep is not just a luxury but a necessary investment in health and wellness, as it's vital for sustaining balance in the body, both physically and mentally. Quality sleep plays a crucial role in cognitive function, affecting memory consolidation, learning, and problem-solving skills. Conversely, deprivation of sleep can result in impaired focus and overall cognitive performance. You may find that if you get too little sleep, processing whatever you've learned during the day can become difficult.

The deep stages of sleep help rejuvenate the body physically. Sleep helps strengthen the immune system, repairs worn-out tissues, and stimulates the release of growth hormones in the body.

How Does Sleep Affect Hormones in the Body?

Sleep affects many hormones in the body, sometimes causing fluctuations in hormonal levels. And in turn, these hormone levels affect your sleep patterns.

Some hormones in the body promote alertness, while others encourage sleep. These hormones work together to create a balanced sleep-wake cycle, known as the circadian rhythm. When there is an imbalance in hormones, you are likely to experience difficulty falling asleep, staying asleep, or waking up feeling energetic.

Getting a good night's sleep is essential for regulating a variety of hormones, including melatonin, cortisol, reproductive hormones like estrogen and progesterone, hunger hormones like leptin, ghrelin, insulin, thyroid hormones, and growth hormones. According to the Sleep Foundation, a lack of sleep can disrupt the aforementioned hormones, leading to imbalances.

Melatonin, the Sleep Hormone

Natural melatonin, the sleep hormone, is the most well-known hormone for impacting sleep. It's an important hormone in regulating your sleep-wake cycle, or circadian rhythm. Melatonin is produced by the pineal gland in the brain. It's released into the bloodstream in response to our exposure to light.

During the day, the level of this hormone remains low, but as the night unfolds, melatonin levels rise, helping us feel sleepy at night and awake during the day. Disruption of sleep and circadian rhythm directly impacts melatonin levels in the body. During the night, especially in the initial stages of sleep, melatonin levels surge, reaching their peak. This nocturnal surge is a testament to the body's readiness for rest and a crucial part of maintaining the circadian rhythms (sleep-wake cycle).

However, exposure to bright light at night or irregular sleep patterns can suppress the production of this hormone, making it harder to fall asleep. In turn, reduced melatonin production may contribute to difficulty falling asleep and maintaining restful sleep, emphasizing the intricate relationship between sleep quality and melatonin release.

Cortisol, the Stress Hormone

Hormones, like cortisol, depend heavily on sleep quality and length for their release. Cortisol exhibits circadian rhythmicity in that its level rises rapidly in the middle of the night and peaks early in the morning, immediately after waking, causing alertness for the activity of the wake cycle.

Several studies suggest that sleeping at night suppresses the release of cortisol. Sleeplessness, on the other hand, is linked to higher hypothalamic-pituitary-adrenal (HPA) activity—the main stress response system—throughout the day, with elevated secretion of cortisol over the latter part of the day instead of its expected fall. This reversal of cortisol's normal rhythm is problematic because it can lead to insulin resistance.

It's highly recommended that you get approximately eight hours of sleep to keep cortisol levels in check.

The Reproductive Hormones, Estrogen and Progesterone—and Thyroid Hormones

Sleep exerts a significant influence on reproductive hormones because in women sleep disruptions can impact the menstrual cycle and fertility.

Lack of sleep can result in abnormally high levels of cortisol for extended periods, which can disrupt the sex hormones. This, in turn, slows the production of your thyroid hormones, which can then affect your metabolism by causing it to slow down.

Leptin, Ghrelin, and Insulin—Hunger Hormones

Poor sleep disrupts these hormones, which are responsible for how food gets metabolized and stored in the body. Inadequate sleep or sleep disturbances can directly affect the production levels of these hormones, which then can cause disruptions to appetite, hunger, and food consumption. This can lead to weight gain. Insulin levels may also be disrupted by poor-quality sleep.

Growth Hormones

Sleep heavily impacts the production of growth hormones in the body. During deep sleep, the body releases this hormone, which plays a vital role in tissue repair and muscle development. Insufficient sleep disturbs this activity, impairing the body's ability to regenerate and rejuvenate itself.

Tips to improve sleep hygiene for better hormonal balance:

- Make your bedroom a sleep-friendly environment (dark, quiet, and cool).

- Establish a regular sleep schedule to regulate your body's internal clock.

- Limit exposure to screens before bedtime, as the blue light emitted can interfere with the production of melatonin, the hormone that regulates sleep.

- Invest in a quality mattress so your body can rest comfortably and deeply.

A Note on Sleep Disorders and Their Impact on Hormones

Conditions like sleep apnea can disrupt hormonal balance. If you have persistent sleep issues, seeking medical advice is important. Treating sleep disorders can help restore hormonal balance and improve overall health.

Zen Zone: Stress Management and Hormonal Health

In today's society, women often juggle diverse roles as caregivers and professionals, balancing family responsibilities with career aspirations and societal expectations. This balancing act places them at the intersection of numerous stressors as they try to navigate the demands of life. There is a pressing need for effective stress-management strategies that address the demands of our daily lives.

What is the relationship between stress and your hormonal health? Chronic stress has the ability to wreak havoc on your hormones as your body continuously releases stress hormones like cortisol. And, as we've seen, high cortisol levels can lead to symptoms like weight gain, fatigue, and mood swings.

The American Institute of Stress highlights that chronic stress can also disrupt the balance of other hormones, affecting everything from digestion to menstrual cycles. In extremely stressful situations, cortisol undergoes an abnormal increase, compromising all other bodily processes.

In the second half of the menstrual cycle, excess production of cortisol can cause the body to produce subsidized amounts of progesterone, which, as a result, can cause estrogen dominance. The combination of less progesterone and more estrogen can impact mood, as progesterone acts as a natural antidepressant. It can also impact fertility, as progesterone stimulates the thickening of the uterine lining for the implantation of an embryo if fertilization occurs.

High levels of cortisol for extended periods of time can contribute to a range of health issues, including disrupted sleep patterns, compromised immune function, and irregularities in metabolic function.

Effective stress management techniques to support hormonal balance:

- Mindfulness and meditation can help regulate stress hormones. Apps like Headspace and Calm offer guided meditations that can help you get started.

- Regular physical activity can also reduce stress levels and help balance hormones.

- Breathing exercises and yoga can help manage stress and support hormonal health.

The Importance of Seeking Help when Stress Feels Overwhelming

Enduring stress for long periods of time can lead to serious problems like anxiety and depression. Recognizing when to seek help because you feel overwhelmed by stress is a crucial step to preserving your mental and emotional health.

Striking a balance in your life through effective stress management helps you break the hold stress has over your life so that you can be happier, healthier, and more productive.

It's essential to seek professional help when stress starts impacting your everyday life. Therapies like cognitive-behavioral therapy (CBT), behavioral therapy, and systemic therapy can provide effective strategies for managing stress and treating symptoms of depression.

Reaching out to loved ones and opening up about stress allows for the exploration of coping strategies, leading to a more balanced life. Numerous non-profit organizations are also available to assist you in addressing the root causes of your stress and providing guidance on how to get better.

Whether it be therapy or confiding in your loved ones, seeking help is a proactive choice that can lead to effective stress management.

Motion Magic: Exercise and Hormonal Health

Regular physical activity can help regulate hormones and improve hormonal health. Moderate exercise can positively impact hormones, notably reducing insulin levels while increasing insulin sensitivity. This allows the body to utilize glucose more effectively, which can help with conditions like PCOS.

Exercise can also help regulate stress hormones, aid in regulating appetite, improve mood, and enhance overall well-being. It can help to decrease excess estrogen levels, improving the symptoms of PMS and other estrogen-dominant conditions. Studies of the PCOS population have also shown that exercise can help improve the regularity and quality of menstrual cycles, contributing to better hormone regulation.

Incorporating regular, gentle exercise into one's routine not only promotes physical fitness but also fosters a hormonal environment conducive to overall health and well-being.

Tips for incorporating exercise into your daily routine:

- Choose activities you enjoy, as you are more likely to stick with them.

- The American Heart Association recommends at least 150 minutes of moderate-intensity exercise each week.

- Make sure to include both aerobic exercises (like walking or cycling) and strength training for best results.

The Impact of Over-Exercising on Hormonal Health

While exercise is beneficial, over-exercising can lead to hormonal imbalances. It's essential to find balance and listen to your body's signals. Over-exercising can lead to changes in the menstrual cycle and decreased bone density, among other issues. If you are experiencing these symptoms, it's important to seek medical advice.

Gut Feeling: The Connection Between Gut Health and Hormones

The gut is home to a vast community of microorganisms, collectively known as the gut microbiome. The gut microbiome houses gut bacteria that are actively involved in the metabolism of hormones, including estrogen, impacting their levels in the body. Poor gut health affects the production of hormones like serotonin, which is produced in the gut. So you can see how the health of your gut is intrinsically linked to your hormonal balance.

Ways to improve gut health for better hormonal balance:

- Include probiotic foods—like yogurt, kefir, and fermented foods—in your diet to support a healthy gut microbiome.

- Eat a variety of high-fiber foods, which can help promote gut health.

- Avoid unnecessary antibiotics, which can disrupt the gut microbiome and impact hormonal balance.

- Eat in a calm and relaxed environment so your body can properly absorb the nutrients you are consuming.

- Avoid inflammatory triggers like refined sugar, alcohol, dairy, and processed foods.

When To Seek Help for Gut Health Issues

If you have persistent gut health issues, seeking medical advice is important. Conditions like irritable bowel syndrome (IBS) and leaky gut can significantly impact hormonal balance and overall health.

Chapter Eight

The Fertility Mystery

Unraveling Hormonal Factors in Fertility and Menopause

If you are currently struggling with being unable to conceive, you are not alone. Millions of people of reproductive age worldwide face the same challenge, with the World Health Organization (WHO) reporting statistics of about 80 million women who have been affected by infertility. Infertility is a condition where you cannot get pregnant after one year (12 months), despite having unprotected sex with the intention to conceive. It's a global health issue, it can affect anyone, and is more common than you might think.

Fertility is known to decline steadily with age. If you're younger than thirty-five, your healthcare provider may diagnose infertility after one year of trying to conceive. However, if you are thirty-five or older, infertility can be diagnosed after six months of regular and unprotected sex.

As women gracefully age, another transformative journey awaits—the transition through menopause. This period, marked by the cessation of menstrual cycles and large shifts in hormones, ushers women into a new phase of life.

In this chapter, we will review how much impact hormonal balance has on fertility and menopause, how to effectively manage these life stages, and how certain factors like nutritional support and stress management may maintain hormone balance and optimize fertility.

Hormonal Harmony: the Key to Fertility

As we all know, hormones play an important role in the development of the female reproductive system and the regulation of the menstrual cycle in women. This goes to show how important hormonal balance is, as it is key to ensuring optimal fertility and reproductive health, guiding the entire process from getting pregnant to perimenopause and menopause. Hormones play a crucial role in ensuring everything works smoothly.

A proper balance of hormones is essential for efficient reproductive health and its functions. Besides aging, certain lifestyle-related factors—like obesity, smoking, alcohol consumption, chronic stress, intense exercise, exposure to environmental pollutants, dietary patterns, and nutritional habits—can exert a negative influence on a woman's fertility.

Infertility can either be primary or secondary. Primary infertility is where a person experiences difficulty conceiving although they have never conceived a child in the past. In secondary infertility, at least one prior pregnancy has been achieved, with the person experiencing difficulties trying to conceive again.

A cross-sectional study of 113 women in the age group of 20 to 35 years, who were experiencing either primary or secondary fertility (57 presented with primary infertility and 56 with secondary fertility), was carried out in the hormone lab of a tertiary care hospital in North India. From the results of this study, it was observed that in primary infertility, a significant positive correlation was observed between serum follicle-stimulating hormone (FSH) levels and other markers of obesity like body weight, hip circumference, and body mass index (BMI). In secondary infertility, serum prolactin and serum thyroid stimulating hormone (TSH) levels also demonstrated a significant positive correlation with body weight and BMI. These findings suggest that there is a relationship between obesity and various hormonal imbalances, which can contribute to infertility.

According to the WHO, an estimated 17.5 percent of the adult population experiences infertility. "Infertility does not discriminate," says Dr. Tedros Adhanom Ghebreyesus, Director-General at WHO (World Health Organization 2023).

About 1 in 5 (22 percent) married couples with a woman aged 30 to 39 experience difficulty conceiving their first child, compared to about 1 in 8 (13 percent) married couples with a woman younger than 30. Fertility diminishes with aging, primarily because egg quality deteriorates over time.

Certain hormones, like estrogen, progesterone, follicle-stimulating hormone (FSH), and luteinizing hormone (LH), work in sync to regulate ovulation and menstrual cycles. An imbalance in these hormones can lead to irregular cycles, making it a challenge to predict ovulation and plan for pregnancy.

Too much luteinizing hormone (LH) is an indicator of infertility. High levels of this hormone in the blood can indicate a decrease in sex steroid hormones from the ovaries, resulting in cases like premature ovarian failure.

An imbalance in the luteinizing hormone and follicle-stimulating hormone (FSH) levels may stimulate excess production of testosterone, which could lead to the common condition of polycystic ovary syndrome (PCOS). Low levels of the luteinizing hormone mean that ovulation does not occur regularly, leading to irregular menstrual periods. Standard LH values for adult women trying to conceive should range from 5 to 25 IU/L. In menopausal women, LH values surge, ranging from 14.2 to 52.3 IU/L.

Prolactin and thyroid-stimulating hormone levels have traditionally been regarded as key components in the examination of infertile women. High prolactin levels, although normal in women or lactating mothers, can interrupt the normal production of the reproductive hormones estrogen and progesterone in non-pregnant women, causing the ovaries to release eggs irregularly or stop altogether.

Normal thyroid stimulating hormone (TSH) levels should be less than 5 mU/l. Greater than 2.5 mU/l is associated with implantation failure and early pregnancy loss. TSH must be at an optimal level, as it affects ovulation. Recent studies have found that TSH should not be higher than 2.5 when trying to conceive; ideally, you want a level between 1 and 2.4 when trying to conceive and 3.0 during pregnancy.

How Do I Maintain Hormonal Balance and Optimize Fertility?

Did you know that reproductive performance can be heavily influenced by food? Nutrition is a major player in maintaining hormonal balance and optimizing fertility. An imbalance in calorie intake and protein intake can be responsible for your being underweight or obese.

Consuming a balanced diet rich in whole foods, lean proteins, and healthy fats can help regulate hormone production and support fertility. For instance, omega-3 fatty acids, found in fatty fish like salmon and mackerel, are known to improve reproductive health by regulating hormone production.

Several studies exploring the effect of various dietary patterns and nutrition on fertility have been carried out over time. These studies use body mass index (BMI) to determine whether an individual is overweight, underweight, or obese. It has been reported and proven that the time to conceive is longer in women with a body mass index (BMI) superior to 25 kg/m2 or inferior to 19 kg/m2, and that both being overweight and obese are significantly related to a reduced fertility rate.

Navigating the Hormonal Seas of Menopause

Menopause represents a significant shift in a woman's hormonal landscape, leading to various symptoms and health concerns. During menopause, the levels of estrogen and progesterone decline, resulting in vasomotor symptoms such as hot flashes, night sweats, mood swings, and sleep disturbances, with about 80 percent of menopausal women experiencing these.

Sleep disturbances, anxiety, and depressive episodes, as well as a decrease in libido and orgasm, are also concerns that come from menopausal changes. If you are nearing the age of menopause or are already menopausal, you are likely to experience various problems if you are negligent toward your health. However, understanding the hormonal changes associated with menopause can help women better navigate menopause and manage symptoms effectively.

Lifestyle modifications can help manage menopausal symptoms and support overall health during this transition. Modifying or limiting unhealthy lifestyle behaviors—like smoking, sedentary lifestyles, and unhealthy diets—helps reduce the risk associated with cardiovascular diseases in postmenopausal women. Postmenopausal women have an increased susceptibility to cardiovascular diseases since estrogen takes a nosedive during this period, which can negatively affect metabolism and cardiovascular health.

Regular physical activity can also help manage weight gain often associated with menopause, improve mood, and promote better sleep. For example, research suggests that practicing yoga can help reduce hot flashes in menopausal women. Cognitive behavior therapy and hypnosis may also improve well-being and decrease the impact of menopausal symptoms.

Nutrition plays a crucial role, too, in managing menopausal symptoms and supporting hormonal balance during menopause. Consuming a diet rich in calcium and vitamin D can help support bone health, as the decline in estrogen levels during menopause can increase the risk of osteoporosis. Foods rich in phytoestrogens, like flaxseeds, soy products, and certain fruits and vegetables, may help balance hormone levels and manage menopausal symptoms.

Although it has not yet been proven in clinical trials, avoiding triggers of vasomotor symptoms like smoking, alcohol, and spicy foods may help you manage your symptoms.

Conventional and Alternative Therapies for Hormone Management

Managing hormones is a complex yet vital aspect of overall health and well-being. Both conventional and alternative therapies are often considered for the relief of menopausal symptoms in middle-aged women.

The reason that up to 70 percent of menopausal women experience vasomotor symptoms, such as hot flashes, is because the hormones driving reproduction cease. Most of the symptoms of menopause are caused by a big drop in estrogen levels, so replacing the estrogen that is lacking in the body is effective in relieving the symptoms of menopause. In the United States, quite a number of women use complementary and alternative therapies, as well as hormone therapy.

Hormone replacement therapy (HRT): This is a common conventional treatment for managing symptoms related to menopause, but it is not suitable for everyone. Doctors may prescribe it to treat hormonal imbalances or inadequate production of hormones following menopause.

HRT involves taking synthetic hormones to replace the declining levels of natural hormones in the body. However, hormone therapy is associated with certain potential risks and side effects, such as breast cancer and endometrial cancer. This makes it essential for women considering these treatments to engage in thorough discussions with their healthcare providers to weigh the pros and cons against the potential drawbacks, as well as exploring alternative approaches that align with their overall health goals.

Estrogen therapy: This is a form of hormone replacement therapy (HRT), and it's quite useful in combating the uncomfortable vasomotor symptoms that often accompany menopause. Although it has proven a bit controversial in the treatment of menopausal women, localized estrogen treatment can sometimes be beneficial in relieving symptoms like itching, dryness, and irritation.

This form of therapy can either be taken orally or transdermally. However, due to the risks associated with estrogen therapy, in cases where there is a definite need for it, the transdermal method of estrogen delivery is preferred to the oral method. This is due to the lower risk of deep vein thrombosis, cholecystitis, osteoporosis, and stroke.

- ***Conjugated estrogens (Premarin):*** derived from the urine of pregnant female horses, this estrogen formulation is a mixture of various estrogens. This form of estrogen is usually taken orally but can also be taken transdermally (by application to the skin or vagina as a cream or by injection into the blood vessel).

- ***Estradiol:*** a bioidentical form of estrogen that is chemically identical to the estrogen produced by the ovaries.

- ***Estropipate (Ogen):*** a synthetic estrogen that is converted into estrone and estradiol in the body. It's available in tablet form and can only be taken orally.

Progesterone/Progestin therapy: Progestins are synthetic forms of the body's naturally occurring hormone, progesterone. Too much estrogen can cause an overgrowth of the endometrium, which can pose a risk to menopausal women in the form of endometrial cancer. These progestins are sometimes used as part of menopausal hormone therapy because they prevent the endometrium from building up too much and becoming cancerous. Examples of progestins include:

- ***Medroxyprogesterone acetate (Provera):*** a synthetic form of progesterone.

- ***Micronized progesterone (Prometrium):*** a bioidentical form of progesterone that is chemically identical to the progesterone produced by the ovaries.

- *Norethindrone acetate:* a synthetic progestin

Combination Therapy: As a result of being highly susceptible to endometrial cancer—particularly in menopausal women taking unopposed estrogen—combined estrogen-progesterone therapy, which involves the co-administration of an estrogen and a progestogen, is usually administered to peri- or menopausal women.

Estrogen-progestin combinations have proved useful in the treatment of moderate-to-severe vasomotor symptoms, vulva and vaginal atrophy associated with menopause, and for the prevention and treatment of osteoporosis (a condition in which your bones become weak). Some combination therapies include:

- *Combination estrogen-progestin products:* Some HRT formulations include a combination of estrogen and progesterone to protect the uterus lining in women with an intact uterus. Examples include:

    - Estradiol and norethindrone acetate (Activella)

    - Estradiol and levonorgestrel (Climara Pro)

    - Conjugated estrogens and medroxyprogesterone acetate (Prempro)

- **Selective estrogen receptor modulators (SERMs):** These are hormone therapies that manage how estrogen works in the body. They are multitaskers. They can either act like estrogen, boosting estrogen levels in your bones to prevent menopausal osteoporosis, or block estrogen from connecting with breast cancer cells to avoid the cells multiplying.

- ***Raloxifene (Evista):*** Although primarily used to prevent and treat osteoporosis, raloxifene has estrogen-like effects on bone and can be considered in postmenopausal women.

- **Testosterone therapy:** In some cases, testosterone may be prescribed as part of HRT for women with low testosterone levels, although this is less common than in men. Menopausal women can often benefit from testosterone therapy.

The normal testosterone range for women is between 15 ng/dL and 70 ng/dL, and if you have less than this in your body around perimenopause and menopause, testosterone replacement therapy can be recommended. Testosterone therapy may help increase sex drive, improve vaginal lubrication, and improve mood and energy.

- **Estratest (esterified estrogens and methyltestosterone):** This is a combination of female sex hormone, estrogen, and testosterone used in the treatment of menopausal symptoms.

- **Bioidentical hormones:** This form of therapy uses processed hormones obtained from plants to mimic the hormones produced by your body. They come in many forms: pills, creams, shots, gels, and implanted pellets.

Like all hormone treatments, there are risks involved. It's highly recommended that you weigh the positives against the negatives with your healthcare provider before commencing this form of therapy, or any type of hormone therapy.

- **Compounded bioidentical hormones:** customized hormone formulations that are often made by compounding pharmacies based on a healthcare provider's prescription. These may include bioidentical forms of estrogen, progesterone, and sometimes testosterone.

There are various alternative therapies available for managing hormonal imbalances related to fertility and menopause. These include herbal remedies, acupuncture, massage therapy, and mind-body practices like yoga and meditation.

For instance, black cohosh and St. John's wort are herbs often used to manage menopausal symptoms. Over-the-counter supplements can also support hormonal balance and manage symptoms related to fertility and menopause.

For example, Vitex (chaste tree berry) is a popular herbal supplement used to regulate menstrual cycles and support fertility.

- ***Black cohosh:*** is widely used to alleviate symptoms of menopause, such as hot flashes and mood swings.

- ***Dong quai:*** Traditionally used in Chinese medicine, dong quai is believed to help regulate the menstrual cycle and ease symptoms of menopause.

- ***Chasteberry (Vitex):*** Known for its potential to balance hormones, chasteberry is often used to alleviate symptoms of premenstrual syndrome (PMS) and regulate the menstrual cycle.

- ***Red clover:*** contains compounds called isoflavones, which may have estrogen-like effects and are sometimes used to manage symptoms of menopause.

- ***Evening primrose oil:*** Rich in gamma-linolenic acid (GLA), evening primrose oil is often used to alleviate symptoms of PMS and support overall hormonal balance.

- *Macafem:* Derived from the root of the maca plant, Macafem is promoted as a natural remedy for hormonal imbalances and menopausal symptoms.

- *Rhodiola:* is an adaptogenic herb that may help the body adapt to stress, potentially benefiting hormonal balance.

- *Ashwagandha:* An adaptogenic herb with potential stress-reducing properties, ashwagandha may help support overall well-being, including hormonal health.

- *Turmeric/Curcumin:* Known for its anti-inflammatory properties, turmeric may help manage inflammation that can impact hormonal balance.

- *Omega-3 Fatty Acids:* Found in fish oil and flaxseed oil, omega-3 fatty acids may help support hormonal balance and reduce inflammation.

- *Calcium and vitamin D:* Important for bone health, these nutrients can be beneficial, especially during menopause, when bone density may decrease.

- *Magnesium:* plays a role in various bodily functions, including hormonal regulation, and may be beneficial for PMS symptoms.

- *B Vitamins:* B vitamins, including B6 and B12, play a role in hormone regulation and may be beneficial for menstrual and hormonal health.

- ***Probiotics:*** are supportive of gut health, and there is emerging research that suggests a connection between gut health and hormonal balance.

However, it's important to consult with a healthcare provider before starting any new supplement regimen.

Chapter Nine

Conquering Hormonal Challenges

A Deep Dive into Endometriosis, PCOS, and Thyroid Issues

Hormonal health challenges are quite common, with many women around the world affected. These hormonal conditions can prove to be quite a challenge, especially for women who want to start a family or conceive.

Polycystic ovary syndrome (PCOS) and thyroid problems share a bidirectional relationship. Research suggests that the same relationship is also evident between endometriosis and thyroid dysfunction. Both syndromes share certain common characteristics and risk factors, such as fatigue, weight changes, mood changes, and hair loss.

The American Thyroid Association (ATA) claims that an estimated 20 million Americans have some form of thyroid disease, with up to 60 percent of those with thyroid disease unaware of their condition. However, although a positive correlation has been observed between these common hormonal challenges, it's important to remember that correlation does not equate to causation. Thyroid issues are linked to a higher risk of the conditions endometriosis and PCOS, but they do not cause them.

To fully understand these hormonal challenges and how to effectively manage them, we will embark on an in-depth journey and exploration of common hormonal health challenges—endometriosis, polycystic ovary syndrome (PCOS), and thyroid issues—and I will help you navigate your way to hormonal balance.

The Hidden Battle: Understanding Endometriosis

Endometriosis is a painful condition where tissue similar to the lining of the uterus is found outside the uterus, causing severe pain, particularly during menstrual periods. It often affects the ovaries, fallopian tubes, and the tissue lining the pelvis. Endometriosis tissue tends to act as the tissue lining the uterus normally would. With each menstrual cycle, endometrial-like tissue thickens, breaks down, and bleeds, resulting in intense discomfort.

This hormonal condition introduces a myriad of challenges, from pain to fertility concerns. "About 25% to 50% of women diagnosed with infertility suffer from some degree of endometriosis," says Dr. Goldstein, MD, and OB/GYN at St. Mary Medical Center.

According to the Endometriosis Foundation of America (2021), endometriosis affects about 1 in 10 women during their reproductive years. Although a handful of factors are thought to increase the risk of endometriosis—like having an immediate family member with the condition, high estrogen levels, a short menstrual cycle, or a heavy menstrual period—it's an idiopathic condition, which means that it has no known cause.

Endometriosis commonly occurs in the lower abdomen or pelvis, but it can also develop in a couple of other places in the body, including the gastrointestinal tract, urinary tract, cervix, bladder, and rectum. The buildup of abnormal tissue outside the uterus can lead to inflammation, scarring, and painful cysts.

The main symptoms of endometriosis are pelvic pain, heavy periods, and fertility problems, but symptoms can vary widely.

Other common symptoms of endometriosis include:

- **Painful sex:** Sex is meant to be enjoyed, not endured. If you encounter pain during or after sex, be sure to consult your healthcare provider, as it may be a sign of endometriosis.

- **Heavy bleeding:** Sometimes, you may experience excessive or irregular bleeding between menstrual periods.

- **Painful bowel movements or urination:** If you observe that you experience pain or difficulty with urination or bowel movements before or during a menstrual period, it's a good idea to consult your healthcare provider, as this is a likely symptom of endometriosis.

- **Infertility:** For some people, endometriosis is first found during tests for infertility treatment.

Other symptoms may include fatigue, diarrhea, nausea, or constipation. These symptoms are usually common on or before your menstrual period.

It's important to note, though, that the level of pain you experience is not dependent on the extent of endometriosis growth in your body. Each person's experience is different. Some people with endometriosis may experience little to no symptoms, only finding out when they find it difficult to conceive. In contrast, for some, they may experience severe and unbearable pain.

How Do I Manage Endometriosis?

There is no cure for endometriosis, but symptoms can be managed effectively. Also, being aware of the symptoms, and whether you could be at higher risk, can help you know when to discuss it with a healthcare provider.

According to the Mayo Clinic (2021), treatment options for endometriosis include painkillers, like paracetamol and anti-inflammatories, and hormone therapy (like the combined pill or the hormonal IUD). Surgery can be used to remove endometriosis and improve fertility, with the most common surgical approach being laparoscopy, also known as key-hole surgery.

Certain dietary changes, like a high-fiber diet, can also help manage symptoms. Regular exercise and stress management techniques, like yoga and meditation, can help manage pain and improve quality of life.

Tests to Check for Endometriosis

Diagnosing endometriosis is a complex process, and healthcare professionals may employ a multidisciplinary approach to ensure a comprehensive evaluation. Your doctor will probably start by performing a physical examination to determine whether you have endometriosis.

Timely intervention and effective management of symptoms associated with endometriosis depend on an early and accurate diagnosis. If you think you might have endometriosis or if you suspect that you might be exhibiting symptoms, it's crucial to speak with a healthcare provider for a comprehensive assessment.

Some of the tests include:

- ***Ultrasound:*** This test uses sound waves to create images of the inside of the body. Ultrasound tests make use of a device called a transducer, which is pressed against the stomach. While a standard ultrasound may not effectively diagnose endometriosis, it can identify cysts linked to the condition.

- ***Laparoscopy:*** This is a minimally invasive surgical procedure to check the inside of your abdomen for signs of endometrial-like tissue. It involves the surgeon inserting a thin viewing instrument with a camera (laparoscope) into the abdomen through a small incision. This allows the surgeon to assess the location, extent, and size of endometriosis growth.

- ***Pelvic examination:*** To check for any unusual changes, your healthcare provider will carry out a pelvic exam on you with one or two gloved fingers. The examination can reveal cysts, irregular growths called nodules, or painful spots that may indicate the presence of endometrial-like tissue in the body.

- ***Magnetic resonance imaging (MRI):*** This is an advanced imaging technique that uses a magnetic field and radio waves to provide crisp images of the organs and tissues in the body. It can help identify endometriomas (cystic lesions) and the extent of the growth. MRI is particularly useful when surgery is being considered, providing the surgeon with detailed information about the location and size of endometriosis growths to plan and guide the procedure.

Knowing the Best Treatment Plan for You

Endometriosis can either be treated with medicine or surgery. Medicine is usually recommended first, with surgery being considered if the medicine does not help with your symptoms.

It's important to work with healthcare professionals to find the best treatment plan for you. Collaborate with doctors, physiotherapists, and dietitians to create a holistic treatment plan. Also, consider joining an endometriosis support group, like the one offered by the Endometriosis Association, for emotional support and shared experiences.

- *Painkillers:* In cases where you may suffer from painful menstrual cramps, your healthcare providers may recommend pain relievers like ibuprofen (Advil, Motrin IB) or naproxen sodium (Aleve).

- *Hormone therapy:* This is also another option your healthcare provider may recommend for you, especially when you are not trying to conceive. Hormone therapy can help ease the pain associated with endometriosis. Although this form of therapy is not a permanent fix, it can help slow the growth of endometrial-like tissue and prevent new growth.

Therapies used in the treatment of endometriosis include:

- *Hormonal contraceptives:* Using hormonal contraceptives may help relieve or get rid of the pain. The primary hormones associated with the development of endometriosis are estrogen and progesterone. Birth control pills, shots, and vaginal rings can help control these hormones, as they tend to stimulate endometriosis.

- *Progestin therapy:* The progestin hormone plays a role in the menstrual cycle and pregnancy. So progestin treatments can stop the growth of endometrial-like tissue and your menstrual periods, which may relieve symptoms. Progestin therapies involve placing a tiny device into the uterus that releases levonorgestrel, a synthetic steroid hormone that is similar to progesterone, or a contraceptive rod placed under the skin of the arm (Nexplanon), or even birth control shots (Depo-Provera).

- ***Aromatase inhibitors:*** These medicines act as inhibitors to help lower the amount of estrogen in the body. It's usually recommended alongside birth control pills or progestin to treat endometriosis.

The Silent Syndrome: Unraveling PCOS

Polycystic ovary syndrome (PCOS) is a common endocrine (hormonal) condition that affects how a woman's ovaries work. This condition can cause multiple ovarian cysts, abnormal hair growth, inflammation, and other symptoms.

A study was carried out on women of childbearing age by the PCOS Awareness Association in 2021. From the study, it was observed that PCOS affects about 1 in 10 women of childbearing age. It's often characterized by irregular periods, high levels of "male hormones," which can cause physical signs like excess facial or body hair, and polycystic ovaries, where the ovaries become enlarged and contain many fluid-filled sacs (The American College of Obstetricians and Gynecologists, 2021).

The signs and symptoms of PCOS include unwanted facial hair or hair growing in a male-like pattern, chronic acne, missed periods, heavy periods, weight gain, and insulin resistance.

How Do I Manage PCOS Symptoms?

Lifestyle modifications can help manage PCOS symptoms and improve quality of life. It's essential, however, to approach these lifestyle modifications with a holistic view. Different individuals respond in different ways to lifestyle changes, so working closely with healthcare professionals, including endocrinologists and gynecologists, is important to developing a tailored approach.

- Regular exercise and a healthy diet can help regulate your menstrual cycle and lower your blood glucose levels.

- In a study by the National University of Natural Medicine in 2020, herbs like cinnamon and turmeric have been found to help manage insulin resistance, a common issue in women with PCOS.

- Weight management is also a key factor in PCOS management. A number of studies demonstrate that if you are overweight, modest weight loss of about 5 to 10 percent of initial body weight improves metabolic, reproductive, and psychological features of PCOS. Achieving and maintaining a healthy weight through the combination of a balanced diet and regular exercise can help regulate menstrual cycles and improve insulin sensitivity.

Medical treatment options for PCOS include birth control pills to regulate menstruation and metformin, often used to treat type 2 diabetes, which manages insulin levels and may prove helpful to some women with PCOS symptoms.

Best Foods to Eat and Avoid for PCOS

Eliminating processed foods, refined sugars, and saturated fats can help people with PCOS prevent complications and set the stage for better long-term health. People with PCOS should avoid the following foods, as they can ramp up inflammation, which is associated with heart disease, as well as raise the risk of other illnesses. Some of these foods include:

- Saturated fats such as margarine and butter
- Red meat
- Carbonated drinks and sugary beverages
- White rice
- Refined foods like white bread, bread rolls, and pasta
- Processed snacks like candy, cookies, and pies

Incorporating non-starchy vegetables and fruits, lean protein, healthy carbs, and low-fat dairy can help make a huge difference in your health and well-being. A Mediterranean diet is highly recommended because it includes fewer ultra-processed foods. It prioritizes foods such as:

- Fresh fruits and vegetables
- Whole grains like brown rice, barley and sorghum
- Protein-rich legumes
- Healthy fats such as olive oil, nuts, and seeds
- Omega-3-rich fish like salmon

The Underestimated Gland: Tackling Thyroid Issues

The thyroid, a small gland in the neck, plays a major role in hormone production and the regulation of various metabolic processes in the body.

Thyroid disorders encompass a wide range of conditions that affect the thyroid gland. According to the American Thyroid Association, thyroid disorders can range from a small, harmless goiter (enlarged gland) to life-threatening cancer, with the cause of these disorders remaining largely unknown.

The most common thyroid disorders involve abnormal production of thyroid hormones: too much (overactivity) of thyroid function causes hyperthyroidism, and too little (underactivity) leads to hypothyroidism.

Symptoms of thyroid disorders can vary widely but often include fatigue, weight changes, mood swings, and changes in menstrual cycles. The American Thyroid Association notes that these symptoms often mimic other conditions, making thyroid disorders difficult to diagnose without proper testing.

Treatment for Thyroid Disorders

This often involves the use of medication to restore normal hormone levels.

- For hypothyroidism, synthetic thyroid hormone levothyroxine is commonly used to supplement deficient hormone levels. (The Mayo Clinic, 2021.)

- For hyperthyroidism, treatments may include radioactive iodine, anti-thyroid medications, or even surgery. Anti-thyroid medications and radioactive iodine treatments are commonly used to reduce the activity of the thyroid gland to normal, with surgical removal of the thyroid gland considered in cases where the aforementioned treatments prove ineffective.

Lifestyle changes, including maintaining a balanced diet and regular exercise, can support overall health and well-being when managing thyroid disorders. Consuming foods rich in nutrients, like iodine and selenium, is particularly important for thyroid health. Iodine, especially, is essential for thyroid hormone production.

Too much stress can throw the endocrine system out of balance, including the hormone levels produced by the thyroid gland. Stress management can positively impact thyroid health. Incorporating techniques like meditation and yoga can help improve the quality of your life.

The British Thyroid Foundation believes that regular exercise can help manage symptoms like fatigue and weight gain associated with thyroid disorders.

Chapter Ten

Your Map to Harmonious Hormones

A Long-Term Plan

"*We are what we repeatedly do. Excellence, then, is not an act, but a habit.*"
– Aristotle

By weaving consistency, certain lifestyle modifications, regular checkups, and exercise into the weft of your daily life, you can sustain hormonal balance over the long run. As you continue on this journey to gaining and maintaining harmonious hormones, let the words of the Greek philosopher Aristotle resonate through your mind.

Aristotle's wise words remind us that excellence—whether in character or hormonal health—is not a fleeting act but a culmination of consistent, healthy, and positive habits. Hormonal health is not achieved through inconsistent efforts but by daily lifestyle choices that you choose to develop.

Choices are made constantly that impact a woman's hormonal health, whether it be a change in dietary patterns, nutrition, sleep, exercise, or stress management. These decisions, over time, tend to shape the foundation for your hormonal health and well-being.

One choice you've made is reading this book, which has helped to equip you with the knowledge and tools you need to maintain hormonal balance over the long run, as well as giving you keys to lasting overall health.

Consistency is Key: the Importance of Routine

Establishing a routine can significantly contribute to hormonal balance. Our bodies love routine, and consistent adherence to healthy practices, such as sticking to regular meal times, a consistent sleep schedule, and a stable exercise regimen, can help regulate hormonal cycles.

Small, consistent changes are often more impactful than larger, less sustainable ones. For example, a fifteen-minute daily walk can be more beneficial for hormonal balance than an intense, one-hour workout once a week.

Consistency in maintaining a balanced diet, rich in hormone-friendly foods, and regularly taking recommended supplements can provide ongoing support for hormonal health. The cumulative impact of these healthy choices, made consistently over time, creates an environment conducive to hormonal harmony.

Regular Check-ups: Stay in Tune with Your Body

Just like any other part of your body, sometimes things can go wrong with your hormones. Being closely in tune with your body will help you notice different symptoms, which, in turn, can help you to identify which hormones are being affected. Regular health check-ups are vital for monitoring hormonal health and catching imbalances early.

Regular appointments for accurate assessment and diagnosis with a trusted healthcare provider, such as Dr. Sara Jane, a renowned women's health practitioner, can help monitor hormonal health over time.

Regular hormonal testing through reputable labs, like ZRT Laboratory, can detect potential imbalances early, allowing for more effective intervention.

Self-monitoring tools, such as the popular hormone tracking app Clue and at-home hormone imbalance tests, can also help you stay aware of changes in your hormonal health.

The Power of Small Changes: Simple Steps for Big Impact

Small, manageable lifestyle changes can have a significant impact on hormonal balance.

Simple dietary swaps—such as replacing refined grains with whole ones, or adding more hormone-balancing foods, like flaxseeds or soy products to your diet—can support hormonal health.

Small adjustments in physical activity, like taking the stairs instead of the elevator, can further help in managing hormonal health over time.

At various points in our lives, we tend to get overwhelmed because life can be stressful. As we know, stress can exert serious repercussions on our health, which is why it's important to make room for mindfulness and rest. Stress management techniques, such as short daily meditation or mindfulness practices using popular apps like Headspace, can help regulate stress hormones and support overall hormonal balance.

Several studies have shown that meditation is a very effective stress management technique. It has been proven to relieve stress after just eight weeks of regular practice. This is because meditation tends to train the mind to be more open, allowing it to more easily cope with life stressors in work, family, finances, school, or relationships.

Nourishment and Rest: the Pillars of Hormonal Health

Proper nutrition and sufficient rest are the fundamental pillars of long-term hormonal health. Cultivating a nourishing approach to diet—one that embraces getting the right balance of key nutrients and mindful eating—enables individuals to make informed and intentional choices about food, fostering an environment conducive to hormonal harmony.

Ensuring your diet is rich in nutrients that support hormonal health, like omega-3 fatty acids and vitamin D, is a simple but powerful way of maintaining hormonal balance.

Regular, restful sleep is also essential for hormonal balance. Strategies to improve sleep quality, such as maintaining a regular sleep schedule and creating a restful sleep environment, can be incredibly beneficial.

Restorative activities like yoga or gentle stretching can help manage stress hormones, too, as well as contribute to overall hormonal balance.

The Journey Continues: Embracing the Ongoing Process

Achieving and maintaining hormonal balance is an ongoing process, not a one-time event. Hormonal health is dynamic and can be influenced by various factors over time, such as aging, stress, and lifestyle changes.

It's important to revisit and adjust your hormonal health plan as your life and body change. This could mean adjusting your diet, exercise routine, or stress management techniques.

Remember to celebrate small victories along the way. Every step you take toward better hormonal health is a win to be acknowledged and celebrated.

Conclusion

In this book we have seen how the endocrine system is a complex network of glands and organs. These glands produce hormones and play key roles in controlling many of the body's activities, such as metabolism, reproduction, growth and development, fertility, stress, and mood. Their influence on our bodies goes much further than we think, even as far as changing how we think and act daily. To live a healthy, high-quality life, we need our hormones to be balanced.

Now that we know quite a bit about how hormones work and the extent to which they affect our lives, it is of utmost importance that we pay close attention to our bodies, recognizing signs of hormonal imbalance early for effective intervention.

Nutrition, lifestyle modifications, exercise, and stress management all play crucial roles in achieving hormonal balance. Maintaining good practices in each of these areas will have a great impact on our many hormonal systems and other aspects of our health.

Do not be afraid to take charge of your hormonal health. While every woman's hormonal journey is different, achieving hormonal balance is possible and can significantly improve the quality of your life. Even common hormonal health difficulties, such as endometriosis, PCOS, and thyroid issues, can be improved in life-changing degrees with proactive measures. Coupled with the knowledge you have gained from this book, consistency, and regular health check-ups, these practices form a robust framework for sustaining long-term hormonal balance.

There is no better time than now to start your journey toward achieving hormonal balance. Try out some of the recipes in this book, start making lifestyle adjustments, and experiment with ways to incorporate the practical tips found in these pages into your daily routine. You can even get started by scheduling a hormone test. Taking these actions will begin to enhance your well-being and contribute to a healthier lifestyle.

As we conclude this beautiful tour into the world of women's hormonal health, I invite you to share your journey, either through email [ashleysullivan818@gmail.com] or on social media [facebook page Dr. Ashley Sullivan, PharmD]. Your experiences and progress are highly invaluable, and we cherish them. Let your stories serve as inspiration to others, and together, we can build a community based on shared experiences and understanding.

From the depths of my heart, I would like to extend my sincere thanks to each of you for the time and dedication you put into improving your hormonal health. I hope that this book has provided you with valuable, credible information and practical strategies for achieving balance in your hormones. And I wish you success on your journey toward hormonal balance. May your journey be transformative and filled with positive changes.

Small Act, Big Impact

Have you ever felt the joy of helping someone just by sharing your thoughts? Leaving a review for "Understanding Hormones for Women" is your chance to do just that! By sharing your experience, you can help others navigate their own hormonal journeys with confidence and clarity.

So, let me ask you this: How amazing would it feel to know that your words could guide someone towards better health and understanding?

Leaving a review is like planting a seed of wisdom. Your insights can blossom into valuable advice for others who are seeking answers about their hormonal health. Plus, it's a fantastic way to reflect on what you've learned and how it's impacted your life.

Why is your review so important? Well, think about the times you've relied on reviews to make decisions. Your honest feedback can be a beacon for someone else, lighting their path towards better health and well-being. It's a small act with a big impact!

Now, here's the fun part – we need your help! If you've enjoyed "Understanding Hormones for Women" and found it helpful, please take a moment to share your thoughts. Your review doesn't have to be long or complicated; just honest and from the heart. Here's how you can do it:

Head over to the book's page on Amazon. Or Click here!
Look for the "Write a Review" section.
Share your thoughts about the book – what you loved, what you learned, and how it helped you. (Bonus points if you include a picture!)
Submit your review and bask in the glow of knowing you've made a difference!

By leaving a review, you're not just helping others; you're contributing to a community of empowered and informed individuals. Your words can inspire someone to take that first step towards understanding their hormones and improving their health.

And here's a little extra motivation – imagine the ripple effect of your review. You're introducing something valuable to someone else, and in turn, you're creating a wave of positivity and goodwill. Other readers and entrepreneurs will appreciate your contribution, and who knows, you might even receive some goodwill in return!

So, let's make a difference together. Share your thoughts on "Understanding Hormones for Women" and help others on their journey towards health and happiness. Thank you for being a part of this wonderful community!

Ways to Connect:

Follow Dr. Ashley Sullivan, PharmD on Facebook, link below
https://www.facebook.com/profile.php?id=100092716005488

Website https://ashleysullivanonline.com/

Join her FREE Facebook group "Compassionate Care and Holistic Advocacy with Dr. Ashley", link below.

https://www.facebook.com/groups/907620087038942

References

Alisa, J., Lynae, R. & Gary, E. (2019, March 14). *Complementary and Alternative Medicine for Menopause.* Journal of Evidence-Based Integrative Medicine.

American Thyroid Association. Retrieved from

Amanda, V. & Tushar, B. (2023, May 22). *Estrogen Therapy.* National Center for Biotechnology Information. Retrieved from

Anne, N., Jill, M. & Miranda, W. (2006, July 24). *Complementary and Alternative Therapies for the Management of Menopause-Related Symptoms:*

A Systematic Evidence Review. Arch Intern Med., 166(14):1453-1465. doi:10.1001/archinte.166.14.1453

Ariane, L. (2023, August 7). *10 Natural Ways to Balance Your Hormones.* Healthline. Retrieved from

Australasian Menopause Society. (2019, May). *Lifestyle and behavioral modifications for menopausal symptoms.* Retrieved from

Aziz-Scott, G. *Hormones and Gut Health: The Importance of Gut Health for Hormone Balance [Blog post].* Retrieved from

Bhavna, S., Sarika, A. & Ritu, S. (2013, February 3). *Association of Obesity with Hormonal Imbalance in Infertility: A Cross-Sectional Study in North Indian Women.* Indian Journal of Clinical Biochemistry, 28(4): 342-347. doi: 10.1007/s12291-013-0301-8

BodyLogicMD. (2023). *Understanding Different Types of Hormone Tests* [Blog post]. Retrieved from

Brody, B. (2023, August 28). *The Endocrine System and Glands of the Human Body* [Blog post]. Retrieved from

Christin, P. (2023, September 19). *How Hormonal Imbalance Can Impact Fertility (And What You Can Do About It)* [Blog post]. Retrieved from

Cleveland Clinic. (2022). *Bioidentical Hormones.* Retrieved from

Cleveland Clinic. *Estriol.* Retrieved from

Cleveland Clinic. (2022, June 6). *Do You Need Hormone Testing?* Retrieved from

Cleveland Clinic. (2022). *Hormones.* Retrieved from

Columbiapsychiatry. (2022, March 16). *How Sleep Deprivation Impacts Mental Health* [Blog post]. Retrieved from

Crystal, E.S., Samantha, M-B. & David, R.R. (2015, February). The Role of Reproductive Hormones in Postpartum Depression. *CNS Spectrums, 20(1), 48-59.* DOI: .

Deborah, B. (2023, August 5). *10 Herbs For Female Hormone Balance.* Integrative Health. Retrieved from

Echelon Health. (2023, November 9). *Understanding Your Female Hormone Profile Results* [Blog post]. Retrieved from

Erica, S., Domenica, L. & Raffaele, P. (2019, June 7). *Nutrition and Female Fertility: An Interdependent Correlation.* Front Endocrinol (Lausanne), 10: 346. doi: 10.3389/fendo.2019.00346

Eleanor, R. (2023, March 6). *What actually happens to your hormones when you exercise?* [Blog post]. Retrieved from

Evangelia, P., Dimitris, E., Evangelos, Z., Codruta, A.P. & Emilia, V. (2022, April 8). *Sleep Deprivation: Effects on Weight Loss and Weight Loss Maintenance.* Nutrients, 14(8): 1549. doi: 10.3390/nu 14081549. Retrieved from

Gabrielle, K. (2023, October 17). *Understanding the Relationship Between Thyroid Function and Endometriosis* [Blog post]. Retrieved from

Gottfried, S. (2020, October 26). *Solutions for a Common Hormone Imbalance.* Retrieved from

Healthline. (2021, July 22). *How Female Hormones Affect Exercise — at Every Age.* Retrieved from

Hey-Ryoung, K. & Hwa-Mi, Y. (2020, November 5). *Facilitators and Inhibitors of Lifestyle Modification and Maintenance of KOREAN Postmenopausal Women: Revealing Conversations from FOCUS Group Interview.* International Journal of Environmental Research and Public Health, 17(21): 8178. doi: 10.3390/ijerph17218178

Hormones' Role on Our Health, and Wellness | Patient Care. (2019). Weillcornell.org; Weill Cornell Medicine. https://weillcornell.org/n ews/hormones%E2%80%99-role-on-our-health-and-wellness

Joanna, G. (2018, September 17). *Prolactin Level Test.* Retrieved from

John Hopkins Medicine. *PCOS Diet.* Retrieved from https://www.hopkinsmedicine.org/health/wellness-and-preventi on/pcos-diet

Kashani L., Nikbakhat, MR. & Akhondzadeh S. (2015, September 16). *Herbal Medicine for Women's Health.* Journal of Medicinal Plants, 14(55).

Kim, Y. M., Seung, D.C. & Aeli, R. (2015, April 27). *Is Complementary and Alternative Therapy Effective for Women in the Cli-*

macteric Period? Journal of Menopausal Medicine, 21(1): 28–35. doi: 10.6118/jmm.2015.21.1.28

LibreTexts Biology. *Types of Hormones - Lipid-Derived, Amino Acid-Derived, and Peptide Hormones.* Retrieved from

Liji, T. (2022, July 7). *Sleep and Hormones* [Blog post]. Retrieved from

Livi. (2022, July 4). *What is body literacy and how can it help you improve your health?* Retrieved from

Mariongluckclinic. *How does Food affect your Hormones?* [Blog post]. Retrieved from

Mariongluckclinic. *Stress and Hormone Imbalance - How to prevent stress from impacting your hormones* [Blog post]. Retrieved from .

Mayo Clinic. (2023, October 12). *Endometriosis.* Retrieved from

Mayo Clinic (2023, September 13). *Infertility.* Retrieved from

McDonald, L. & Helms, E. (2018). *The Women's Book: Volume 1. A Guide to Nutrition, Fat Loss, and Muscle Gain.* Austin, Texas: Lyle McDonald Publishing

Meissner, H.O., Mscisz, A., Reich-Bilinska, H., Kapczynski, W., Mrozikiewicz, P., Bobkiewicz-Kozlowska, T., Kedzia,B., Lowicka, A., Barchia, I. (2006, December). *Hormone-Balancing Effect of Pre-Gelatinized Organic Maca (Lepidium peruvianum Chacon): (II) Physiological and Symptomatic Responses of Early-Postmenopausal Women to Standardized doses of Maca in Double Blind, Randomized, Placebo-Controlled, Multi-Centre Clinical Study.* Int J Biomed Sci, 2(4):360-74. Retrieved from

Ningthoujam, N. (2023, October 17).

Cruciferous vegetables: Nutritious foods you need to balance hormones [Blog Post]. Retrieved from

Northwell Health. (2018, November 27). *11 unexpected signs of hormonal imbalance.* Retrieved from

Pensacola Wellness. (2018, February 21). *How Nutrition affects your Hormones* [Blog Post]. Retrieved from

Rajiv, S., Yashdeep, G., Manju, K., & Sameer, A. (2015). *Thyroid disorders and polycystic ovary syndrome: An emerging relationship.* Indian Journal of

Endocrinology and Metabolism, 19(1): 25–29. DOI:

Robert Lustig Website | Promoting global metabolic health and nutrition. (n.d.). (2024) Robertlustig.com. https://robertlustig.com/

Rootfunctionalmedicine. (2023, October 31). *Foods that Help Balance Hormones* [Blog Post]. Retrieved from

Shams T, Setia MS, Hemmings R, et al. Efficacy of black cohosh-containing preparations on menopausal symptoms: a meta-analysis. 2010. In: Database of Abstracts of Reviews of Effects (DARE): Quality-assessed Reviews [Internet]. York (UK): Centre for Reviews and Dissemination (UK); 1995-. Available from:

The Link Between Hormones and Mental Health. (2024). (n.d.). Verywell Mind. https://www.verywellmind.com/the-link-between-hormones-and-mental-health-7500077#:~:text=%E2%80%9CHormones%20can%20have%20a%20big%20impact%20on%20your

Trinity Health Mid-Atlantic. (2023, March 27). *Overcoming two common fertility problems* [Blog post]. Retrieved from

Veronica, D. & Nicholas, P. (2022, May). *Alternative and non-hormonal treatments to symptoms of menopause.* Best Practice & Research Clinical Obstetrics & Gynaecology Volume 81:45-60. Retrieved from

Weill Cornell Medicine. (2020, December 17). *Hormones' Role on Our Health, and Wellness.* Retrieved from

Wendy, W. (2023, June 5). *The Link Between Hormones and Mental Health.* VerywellMind. Retrieved from

World Health Organization. (2023, April 4). *1 in 6 people globally affected by infertility: WHO.* Retrieved from

www.ingramcontent.com/pod-product-compliance
Lightning Source LLC
Chambersburg PA
CBHW070611030426
42337CB00020B/3757